HOW TO HELP YOUR MAN LOSE WEIGHT

A GUIDE FOR THE CONCERNED WOMAN

Jerry C. Sutkamp, M.D.

and

Ted Mason

SIMON & SCHUSTER
NEW YORK • LONDON • TORONTO • SYDNEY • TOKYO • SINGAPORE

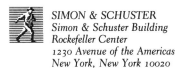 SIMON & SCHUSTER
Simon & Schuster Building
Rockefeller Center
1230 Avenue of the Americas
New York, New York 10020

10 9 8 7 6 5 4 3 2 1

Library of Congress Cataloging-in-Publication Data
is available
ISBN 0-671-74455-0

All personal (before) photos courtesy of the
individuals. All professional (after) photos courtesy
of Physicians Weight Loss Centers.®

Although this book provides a specific diet, Dr. Sutkamp, National Medical Director of Physicians Weight Loss Centers of America, Inc., highly recommends a full-service weight-loss program that includes medical screening, behavior modification, an effective weight loss/maintenance agenda, and an exercise component, such as Physicians Weight Loss Centers offers.

Although this book provides a specific diet, Dr. Sutkamp, National Medical Director of Physicians Weight Loss Centers of America, Inc., highly recommends a full-service weight-loss program that includes medical screening, behavior modification, an effective weight loss/maintenance agenda, and an exercise component, such as Physicians Weight Loss Centers offers.

Acknowledgments

The list of those who helped bring *How to Help Your Man Lose Weight* from interesting idea to bound book is a long one, but the authors want to express their gratitude to those who were especially helpful. Susanne Jaffe, our editor at Simon & Schuster, knew a good thing when she saw it and displayed unerring editorial sense across the board. The same could be said of Barbara Lowenstein, the literary agent who brought us to Susanne. Charles Sekeres, Cliff Kocian, and Cynthia Konstand of Physicians Weight Loss Centers, had faith that this would be a different kind of weight-loss book even when it was in the planning stage. Robert L. Green provided the spark that sent us forward, while Dan Curtis, R.D., and Matt Segal were a godsend in formulating a diet that men could live with and *like*. And Dr. George Bray, of UCLA, has made a new perspective on obesity possible with his pioneering research. Most importantly, I would like to thank all the obese men and women patients I've treated in the past twenty-five years who have inspired me to learn as much as possible about their physical and psychological problems associated with their disease.

Contents

8   CONTENTS

Author's Note

How to Help Your Man Lose Weight: A Guide for the Concerned Woman is a book designed to assist women in helping men to lose weight in a practical, no-nonsense way that works.

If you're anxious to get on to the purely practical sections of the text regarding food and exercise, I will ask you for a little patience. I spend a good deal of time talking about the root causes of male overweight in the opening chapters (as well as your role in his weight loss), and I think that it's important for you to understand *why* he's fat and *how* he sees his weight—and yours—before you can really begin to help him help himself.

I've also provided pictures of men from around the country who've managed to defeat their weight problem, following the Physicians Weight Loss Centers® principles. They provide useful inspiration—for you and for him—and proof that it can be done.

As for the practical, although a 30-day meal plan is provided, I don't consider this a "diet book" as such: The plan is meant more to provide guidance on how meal-planning can be rethought with his taste, his waist, and your budget in mind. I expect that you'll be adding your own recipes and new finds at the market well before the first thirty days are up. Nothing in the plan is written in stone—except that he should have no more than 30% calories from fat during the course of a given day. But take note of the balance of the basic food groups in each daily menu, and remember that the plan was formulated with nutrition as well as fat content in mind.

The walking chapter is a little less changeable; he's got to hit the pavement once a day on a regular basis or it'll take him quite a bit longer to drop his unwanted pounds.

How to Help Your Man Lose Weight: A Guide for the Concerned Woman is what I've found diet and weight loss books *not* to be since I started working with overweight men: *it's do-able,* and if both of you make the changes I recommend, it'll have a lasting effect on your lives. I wrote it to take peoples' minds off womens' weight for once, and focus attention on how the other half of society—men—can be awakened to the dangers of overweight. Once you've helped him see the light, let's have a little faith that the switch will stay on.

JERRY C. SUTKAMP, M.D.

INTRODUCTION

Why a Book About Overweight Men— for Women?

American men are a stubborn bunch when it comes to taking advice; they won't listen to you even when what you're trying to tell them is for their own good. They're particularly deaf when it comes to listening to the wisdom of other men, especially doctors. The women in their life, though, seem to be better at getting men to do what's good for themselves.

That's why, after almost twenty years of treating obesity and the problems it causes, and having very little luck in getting overweight men into my office before they get really sick, I decided to write a book about men and their weight *for women to read and use.* A woman, be she mother, wife, girlfriend, daughter, sister, or just good neighbor, is often the closest person to a particular overweight man. She sees him most often, she knows his strengths and weaknesses—and she has greater influence on his behavior than anyone else in his life.

It's also the right time for this book, in terms of the medical community and the food industry. As doctors, we now know more than ever before about the medical consequences of fat, the role of other substances in weight gain, and how exercise should be incorporated into any weight-loss program. We also know more about the differences between the sexes than we did even a decade ago. And, thankfully, the food industry has begun to respond to consumer demand for more healthful foods that don't taste like birdseed.

I first realized how much influence a woman can have over the eating habits and general behavior of her man when I started trying to get some of the overweight guys who were living with women patients of mine to come into my office. They'd usually drive their wife, daughter, or girlfriend to my clinic, and as soon as they climbed out from behind the wheel, I could see that they should be on a weight-loss program themselves. Having another overeater in the house when you're trying to lose a few pounds yourself makes the job twice as difficult (it's a little like a recovering alcoholic living and working in a well-stocked bar), so I'd try to talk to them in a friendly way about starting a weight-loss program. Here's a little sample of how most of those conversations went.

> Gosh, George, good to see you. Looks like you put on a few pounds. Have you thought about joining Marilyn and losing some weight yourself?
>
> (Pained look, nervous or irritated tone) Nah, Doc—I've always been kind of a big guy. . . . Honey, you just about ready to go?

Then there'd be a quick exit. After that, you can bet that he'd wait outside in the car rather than talk to me. The tone may have varied slightly (white-collar and professional men tended to dismiss me as if I were a junior salesman who'd said something stupid, while working guys would more often make a joke out of what I'd said), but the I-don't-know-and-I-don't-want-to-know attitude was the same across the board.

More out of curiosity than anything else, I started talking to women in my clinic who were involved with overweight men, about the potential health risks and early death that "big guys" faced because of their weight; about the damage they were doing to them-selves and their loved ones—and how most men seemed completely unaware that too much body fat is just as big a problem for males (bigger, in some ways) as it is for females.

Surprisingly, a lot of the women I spoke to hadn't thought about men and fat much, either. They were used to thinking of themselves and other women as having weight problems, not their men. Even though most of the women I dealt with weren't exactly happy that those svelte Prince Charmings they once knew had started to look like Henry VIII sinking his teeth into the nearest wild boar, they didn't think of their men as having a health problem. This was true despite the fact that some of these guys probably wheezed and rattled after going up a flight of stairs and couldn't get into the suit jackets they'd had the tailor let out just a year ago.

I decided to try a little experiment. Where my take-the-bull-by-the-horns approach had failed, I decided to work with my women patients to try to get their overweight men to slim down. We made use of the control most of them had over the food in the house and of their strong influence on their men's leisure-time activities. In general, I asked each woman to take what she'd learned from the program we'd developed at Physician's Weight Loss Centers (of which I'm national medical director) about eating, eating habits, and exercise, and teach it to her man.

The program we put in place didn't involve "talking" to him or just trying to put saccharine instead of sugar on the dining-room table. I'd been an overweight man myself and I'd treated overweight people for too long to believe that either method would work, with men or women. I was asking a woman to help her man change his behavior—no easy task. But through the course of treating almost a million patients, I'd learned that only by addressing the whole person does a weight-loss campaign succeed. In this case, though, I needed the help of someone who was central to the man's life, who understood weight gain and loss, and who could also exert *control* and *influence* over his diet.

With my help, several of my women patients set to work to help their men lose weight. There were ten slightly porcine males in this first group with an age range from thirty-three to sixty-one. The youngest had just a bit of a gut to lose—about fifteen pounds; the others were from 30 to 40 pounds on the wrong side of the scale. By far the 30 to 40 pounders are more common among men.

I considered dealing with their men's weight as helpful to the women as well, since it's very difficult to maintain your newfound thinness when you're constantly around a partner who overeats and who subtly (or not so subtly) tries to get you to do the same. Studies, such as one conducted at Purdue University in Indiana a couple of years ago, show that having a partner trying to lose weight along with you makes long-term, healthy weight maintenance easier and success more likely.

The results of my little experiment were pretty good: eight of the men did lose, and many got back to the weight they were when they were much, much younger. In some cases, they never knew their eating habits had been changed for them. In others, they took credit for the positive changes in their lifestyle themselves—especially if any kind of new athletic prowess (like being able to walk four blocks without stopping to catch breath) resulted. But the end product was the same: thinner men who were more likely to lead longer, healthier lives. My conclusion: successful weight loss in a man depends in large measure on the woman in his life.

This took place a few years ago. In the 1990s, the task of changing a man's weight has been made easier for a number of reasons. We now know much more about the role of fat (versus calories alone) than we did before 1988, after the surgeon general warned us to get the fat in our diets below 30 percent. Complex carbohydrate foods like pasta and potatoes are now recognized for their important role in weight loss. We know that upper body fat (where men pack it on) is different from lower body fat. Instead of trying to jog our pounds away as we did in the early 1980s, university research of the last few years has shown that walking beats any other kind of exercise in strengthening the heart and bringing our weight to a healthy level—and believe me, it's a lot easier to get a man to walk than to run.

Best of all, after many years of ignoring the problems that unhealthy foods have created for American men and women, the food industry has responded to our desire for the taste of fat and sugar—but recognized our need to get the fat out of our lives. New cuts of beef and pork, skinless chicken and turkey, alternate low-fat and nonfat toppings and other condiments, good-tasting sugar substitutes—a whole slew of high-quality, low-fat grocery products that replace dangerous male favorites (like butter and mayonnaise) has hit the shelves just in the past two years. Even McDonald's has joined the low-fat parade. That's good news and it's important news when you're dealing with male eating habits.

Now, I'm not promising that if you have a Jack Bow-legs in your life, he's going to turn into Kevin Costner overnight if you follow my suggestions. Results will vary from man to man. But he will be a much-improved specimen, I can promise you that. Not just to look at either, but to live with. Bad eating and drinking habits and excess weight often result in the couch potato-ism and sullen male behavior that drive women crazy.

What I have realized during my years dealing with overweight people is that women already have the essential tools they need to help men close to them lose weight. They usually buy the groceries or decide what's bought, and they also have a great deal to say about what their men do with their spare time. What they *don't* have is a clear understanding of how men think about their excess baggage and how they got to think that way. It's that understanding, along with a healthy diet and exercise program, that I want to communicate to you with this book—as well as a vision of how your man's weight loss can change you, him, and your life together.

How to Help Your Man Lose Weight is for you if you have an overweight man in your life, whether he's a relative, friend, husband, lover, roommate, or son who hasn't left the nest yet; whether he's been that way for a long time or whether he's just started packing on the pounds. And you don't have to have a weight problem yourself to be able to help him with his.

My book takes the same approach as my weight-loss treatments: to improve the whole, you have to have an understanding of the parts, both body and mind. That's especially true when you're talking about men and weight.

PART ONE

THE OVERWEIGHT MAN

CHAPTER ONE

Saddlebags vs. Love Handles: How a Man Gains, Carries, and Loses Weight Differently from You

Why is it we never seem to notice overweight men as much as overweight women? That's a question I asked myself a few years back, when I was stuck in a midwestern airport for a couple of hours waiting for a connection.

As a bariatric physician, my practice revolves around people and their weight, so I was in the snack bar watching the crowd instead of reading my medical journals, as I should have been. One couple in particular caught my eye. He was in his mid- to late-thirties and she was about the same age. They had the sort of comfortable look you get from being together for a few years, so I assumed they were a couple. But where she'd pretty much kept her figure, he was about 30 to 40 pounds overweight—not huge, but uncomfortably big, and out of shape to boot. You could see that he'd been a good-looking guy, but now he was showing all the signs that would probably bring him into an emergency room with a heart attack in a few years. He was breathing hard from carrying their luggage just a little ways, his skin had an unhealthy pale sheen to it, and his shirt buttons were popping out from all the weight around his belly and chest. But then came the capper: When they sat down across from me, she stayed and watched the bags while he went and got a Diet Coke for her—and two hot dogs for himself. She was the thin one, being careful about what she ate, while he wolfed down that fatty meat as if he could still get into a 30-inch pair of jeans.

Watching those two, I got to thinking about all the patients with weight problems that I'd treated since the early 1970s—about 90 percent of them were women. I knew that at least as many men as women had a weight problem—the proportions, in fact, are just about even. Of the 65 million people in the United States who can be considered unhealthfully overweight (those who are 20 percent or more above their ideal body weight) just about half of them are men. Take these figures just a little bit further and they tell you that almost *one-quarter* of adult men and an equal number of adult women should lose some excess baggage if they want to stay healthy. What's more, I knew from treating a few men that overeating can cause more serious health problems for them than for women, and that diets that work for women usually don't work for men. I started wondering why, with everything we know in the 1990s about the problems that too much weight can cause, I never see the husbands and boyfriends until they have life-threatening problems like diabetes or heart disease and are forced to lose weight if they want to stay alive. Sometimes they're successful, sometimes not. A man pays in a thousand different ways for his big gut and his love handles—on the job, in his relationships, at the doctor's office. But there was my friend at the airport, chomping away on all that fat and sodium.

What I realized was that men don't seek help for weight problems not only because they're *physically* different from women in the ways they gain and carry weight, but they're also *psychologically* different in their attitude toward weight and weight problems. It's a dangerous combination; they know less and think less about the costs of excess pounds than you do, and by ignoring the problem they make it worse.

An overweight man doesn't pay the cost alone. As the woman in his life, and as his partner, you pay as well. A man has become overweight since you've known him has not only changed physically. He's now different in his attitude toward you, toward his children, toward his job. He's also well on his way to developing weight-related conditions that will shorten his life by a dozen or more years—at least.

My own weight has long been a problem for me, and I realized early on what an important role my wife had played while I was losing. She was both partner and drill sergeant. But I also realized that I'd been more honest with myself and with her about my spare tire than most men are, and my admission helped her to help me. I filled her in on what my problem eating areas were—and they were a lot different than hers or any other woman's, as they are for most men. Most men can't or won't talk about their own weight with women, though, and they're uncomfortable talking about it with other men. They just don't know how.

It doesn't have to be your mate who has the problem, either, for you to take action. With more adult sons living at home than ever before (about 30 percent of the single males aged twenty-five to thirty-four, according to a recent *New York Times* study), and with women in charge of shopping and preparing meals for a variety of males in a wide variety of domestic situations, knowledge of food and male eating habits is more important than ever before.

MEN WHO EAT TOO MUCH

I've never known a man to show any guilt at all about eating what he wants, when he wants it—no matter how fat he is. Men are completely unself-conscious about their eating habits, and don't care who sees them downing enough food for an elephant—in fact, I sometimes think they like having other people see how much they can eat. Women, on the other hand, have been taught since childhood to be self-conscious about what and how much they eat. The differences aren't only in attitude, but in eating *patterns*. If you've ever been curious about how a man gains so much weight when he runs past you without eating a morning meal and you've prepared his dinner, listen to Peggy Henderson, who finally got her husband, Tom (he was thirty-seven, 5'10", weighed 275 pounds and had one heart attack under his belt) to come see me.

PEGGY

Tom used to leave the house in the morning without eating a thing, so I wondered how he was getting so big, because he didn't eat more than usual for dinner. Then I found out he was stopping at the coffee shop in the morning and buying a dozen chocolate-covered donut holes every day—those cheap little things that aren't even a real donut. And you know *how* I found out? He was eating them while he was driving along so he wouldn't have to share them when he got to work, and while he was chasing one that rolled across the front seat he ran into a telephone pole.

Peggy's story has an unusual ending (Tom wasn't hurt), but the circumstances are pretty typical. A man will often skip breakfast, but stop on the way to work, pick up a bag of donuts or some other junk food. Then he'll often eat far more than necessary at lunch—for you, it would be a major meal. A sugary snack at about four o'clock in the afternoon results in him gobbling a huge dinner (more on sugar's role in men's weight in Chapter 6). And men do *gobble* food—lots of it—whenever they eat, but especially at dinner. Women don't. Even if they have a weight problem, women don't wolf down food the way men do. They tend to eat smaller portions more frequently throughout the day, and to snack more. Men rarely cook the food they eat; it's either beer or burgers (or both) or you make it for him.

THE MALE DIETER

When you're talking about men and weight loss, *it's important to remember that men need a diet that doesn't seem like a diet.* I've found that they're just not as adaptable to new foods as you are. They have to have an eating plan with a lot of protein (the new lean meats can provide it) and they'll basically want to keep on eating as though they're not doing anything special. One of my weight-loss patients (he went from 230 to 165 pounds), Bob Hughes, had this to say about a prior, unsuccessful attempt at reduction, and I think it applies to almost all men who try to lose.

> The first time I tried a diet, some crazy book had my wife mixing and matching different food groups and me eating tofu instead of meat—she wouldn't even let me have a piece of chicken. I didn't even know what tofu *was*. It lasted about a week before I went back to my regular steak and potatoes with gravy. I went to the market myself and brought the food back. I'm not really much good with a stove, so my wife finally gave up and cooked it for me.

The cornerstone of a successful weight-loss program for men lies in duplicating their traditional eating habits—but with far less fat and sugar—and with getting them to exercise. You've got to have both. Cottage cheese just won't do the trick, whether a man is a day laborer or a CEO. Since, for better or worse, most women still control the kitchen and what goes into it (men don't think about *groceries*, they think about *food*), you play an important role in making sure he sticks to foods that both satisfy him and help him to lose.

HOW FAT IS HE?

In every doctor's office and in every gym and weight-loss clinic across the country, you'll come across a chart from the Metropolitan Life Insurance Company that's been in use for over thirty years, giving "desirable" weights for men and women, according to their frame size (small, medium, large) and their height.

Sounds good, and in general these charts are of some use as a general reference. The problem is, there are *lots* of exceptions to the chart recommendations, among both men and women. Rarely is a person one body type from head to toe (that's why most physicians don't even like to use the body-type labels endomorph, mesomorph, and ectomorph when referring to body shape anymore). Ethnic origins vary, and that affects your height and weight. And since the chart was meant to assess people for life insurance, the men and women it measures tended to be typical Americans—slightly overweight. To top it all off, studies done at Harvard show that people with a body weight 10 percent *below* the ideal weights listed in the chart have the lowest death rates in the country.

These charts don't show you what percentage of body *fat* a man or woman has, and that's a very important factor, when you're figuring out how overweight someone is. An example: If a solid-muscle football player goes in to be weighed, he'll often be pronounced overweight according to the Metropolitan Life weight chart when in fact he's in tip-top shape, and probably has less than 15 percent body fat. A good goal for your average man is 15 to 20 percent body fat. For women, about 10 percent higher is okay.

THE EYEBALL AND EAR TESTS

Frankly, though, it's not that easy to get a pair of calipers around a portion of your man's skin to find out his percentage of body fat. I'd vote for the eyeball and ear tests instead. You can tell when he's fat and when he's not by looking at him and then by listening to how he breathes after he's climbed a flight of stairs. And if you have any doubts, be your own set of calipers. Reach over and try to pinch a fold of flesh together between your fingers just above his belt line. If you can get more than an inch between your fingers, you should keep reading.

MALE AND FEMALE WEIGHT LOSS

Many of the women I've counseled on how to get their man to lose weight become frustrated because men lose faster than women. They often assume that their own situation is unique, which is wrong from the get-go because men and women have distinctive characteristics when it comes to weight gain and loss. So it's a good idea to start with a basic knowledge of the overall gain/lose differences between the sexes.

The only thing that's the same for both of you is the yo-yo dieting factor: According to our National Institutes of Health in Bethesda, Maryland, 95 percent of men *and* women regain the weight lost in fad diets within two years. And of that 95 percent, a startling number gain back all their old weight *plus* a few extra pounds.

Then we come to the physical differences. Men gain most of their weight around the chest and stomach, whereas you will put it on around the thighs, backs of the arms, and buttocks. It's an important difference; all his flab is around vital organs (especially the heart) where it squeezes in and causes serious medical complications for him.

The male weight condition I'm describing in this book doesn't really apply to men who've had a weight problem since they were boys. Their numbers are fairly small, and men who were overweight as youngsters tend to be as conscious of their weight as you are. They also tend to do something about it at an earlier age, and they tend to seek help on their own. So the men I'm talking about started having a weight problem at a relatively late age, compared to women. It usually started gathering steam when they were about thirty.

Most men who have had an obesity problem from an early age have a unique body type. Their overweight is called *gynoid* (the pounds are packed around the hips and backside), as opposed to the *android* shape that most men have (the weight's around the upper body). The gynoid male is one who's shaped like a pear, tends to waddle when he walks, and he usually dresses in sweatsuits or other sacklike clothes because he has a hard time finding anything else that will fit. Often, his skin is almost fine or hairless. Because he has often been overweight in the same places women are, he tends to be much more knowledgeable about dieting and exercise than other men. He also tends to be much more empathetic about women's weight problems because he's been there himself. But, even though a gynoid man will never have a V-shaped body, he can keep his weight down and his body in decent proportion.

Gynoid men have the toughest row to hoe psychologically when it comes to coping with their fat because, basically, they are shaped like women. They tend to be extremely self-conscious about their hips and thighs, and are very much aware of the fact that they're overweight. But, as you'll see shortly, the placement of extra weight on their lower body is actually an advantage, since they don't have the health problems that fat around the chest area causes in other men.

Barrel-chested men outnumber their bell-bottomed brothers by about ten to one, so most women are more familiar with men who have upper-body weight problems. The major psychological difference between the two types? Gynoid men expect too much of weight-loss programs at an early age, while android men are willing to do too little about their weight at any age.

Some of the medical facts about men, women, and dieting will make you even angrier if you've ever battled a weight problem of your own: you have a higher percentage of body fat (about 10 percent higher, in fact) than your man, regardless of whether he's overweight, and your overall calorie-burning capability is about 10 percent *lower*. His metabolism will remain about 10 percent faster than yours, typically, throughout your lives.

The upshot of all this is that if your husband is your same relative age and weight, and the two of you sit across the table from each other and go fork-to-fork over the same plate of food, you'll gain weight and he won't. And no matter what kind of diet it is, if you're both on it, he can lose 4 pounds to your 3 pounds in two weeks. It can be pretty frustrating. Listen to a patient of mine, Rebecca Simmons, who tried a fad diet herself before she came to me:

> I remember my boyfriend, Dennis, when I went on this weird diet—liquid food and stuff. He made me look like Slenderella, with his big gut. Well, wouldn't you know that *he* was the one who started losing, just because he was used to raiding my icebox and the only thing in it now was the diet formula. I lost 6 pounds, but he lost 10. Then he got tired of it and started going down to the store himself for ice cream. We both gained all the weight back in just a couple of weeks.

Rebecca's case illustrates many things about a relationship that revolves around weight and food that I'll talk about in depth later: the sabotage of an improvement program by a mate; the resentment that grows when one partner loses (in this case by accident) and the other doesn't; and men who eat for emotional reasons. But the most important fact for you to know is a genetic one: men will always lose faster than women, and if you have a weight problem yourself, you shouldn't think that he has more willpower than you do—it's just nature's way.

WHEN DO MALE WEIGHT PROBLEMS START?

Women start out with an age/weight disadvantage compared to men. While you were confronting your first date and getting braces, that's probably when you started to be conscious of your weight as well. Adult men didn't have the same problem. In fact, most adolescent boys are far more concerned about *gaining* weight than losing it, since they've already learned to associate size with power—a belief that will cause them problems later, as their quarterback's shoulders start dropping toward their waist.

Men start to have weight problems when their metabolism slows down and when years of self-indulgent eating and drinking habits begin to catch up with them. That's one of the important reasons grown men are so oblivious to the fact that they're overweight; they've just never had to give it a thought before. In their late twenties they begin to gain; in their late thirties and early forties, they really pack it on. Up to age forty, men have a 12 percent chance of being obese; after forty, it jumps to 38 percent; that's 10 percent higher than the risk for you.

Proportionally, too, men are just as overweight for their size as women are, after they reach age thirty. Age thirty is a magic number when you're dealing with men and weight. Not only are 25 percent of men without a good part of their hair by then, but the same number are in sad physical shape.

Statistics aside, stress begins to affect men as well. Because men are so emotionally bottled up, they begin to look to food as a kind of sedative. On the other hand, sometimes they just like to make pigs of themselves.

DIETS THAT DON'T WORK

Even if your man were ready and willing to head into the nearest diet clinic (he probably isn't), a program there that might work for you isn't likely to work for him. Our national obsession with weight loss over the past few years has resulted in the opening of thousands of nonmedical weight-loss clinics and the sale of millions of expensive canisters of powders, potions, and other magic formulas all promising the quickest road to Thin heaven. In general, you can assume that these Band-Aid solutions will work for a limited time with women (usually about a year, but no longer than two before the weight returns), but they're definitely not designed with a man in mind.

Because men are generally larger and heavier than women, even when they're not overweight, they need more calories and protein to function normally and maintain optimal health. Whereas the *average* (not dieting) woman takes in about 1,300 to 1,500 calories per day, the average man consumes about 2,000 to 2,500. When a woman places herself on the 800- to 1,200-calorie-a-day program that most diets call for, she's going to find it rough going, at least for a while. But take a man and place him on that same program without any adjustment for his different physical needs, and he's going to be cheating in half the time that she is—he's twice as hungry!

Psychologically, men are ill-equipped for diets that might work for women. Men are used to eating big meals at specified times, and to suddenly replace that with a half-meal—or worse yet, some powder and milk—will result in their going back to old habits in pretty short order. And men feel self-conscious going to diet centers or participating in any kind of group program—especially if most of the group is female.

In the work world, the last thing that men want other men to know is that they're on a "diet." Diets are perceived to be feminine. A man on a diet is admitting he has a "weakness," and you'll find that most men would rather blow up like a blimp and have a dozen coronary bypasses before they'll admit to being needy in front of

other men. Can you picture an executive at lunch with his staff pulling out a packet of powder and asking for a tall glass of nonfat milk and a spoon? Just the thought's enough to give most men a heart attack.

Forty-four-year-old Ed Henshaw, a lawyer at a Fortune 500 company near my clinic, was one of my few male patients. He was severely obese at 5′11″, 275 pounds, and didn't have much choice except to come to me—he had all the early signs of weight-related diabetes. His first male weight-loss/business lunch experience is pretty typical:

> We were at a very expensive steakhouse in town, a classic businessmen's watering hole. When I ordered a Caesar salad and a mineral water you could have heard a pin drop. For a minute I almost gave in and ordered some prime rib, but I didn't want to end up in the hospital again. Then the jokes started—usually revolving around bird food and Volkswagen buses and life on the commune. At least half the men at that table should've lost a few pounds and I think they felt threatened. But if I'd hadn't been in poor health because of my weight, I don't know if I could have faced them down.

Women, on the other hand, have a greater sense of community and are more willing to extend support to other women in discussions about their weight problems and general health. Unlike men, they don't view owning up to a weight problem—or any problem—as presenting someone else with an opportunity to do them dirt. They make diets a regular subject of conversation. When women are out to lunch in a group, they'll often make a point of discussing the low-cal, low-fat fare they've ordered—perhaps a little too much. But men don't do it enough.

MEN AND POWDERED "MEALS"

It's strange, but I've found that a lot of men who are conscious of the need to lose (they're in the minority) will try to use so-called liquid meals in private and not tell anyone they're on them. Whereas most men have no qualms about wolfing down a steak and potatoes slathered with butter and sour cream, they don't want to be seen drinking a milkshake.

Although going on a liquid diet—it's fasting, really, because there is no such thing as a "replacement" for a well-balanced meal—is a bad idea for both men and women, in my experience these products fail more quickly, and more dangerously, with men than with women.

In general, men will do "better" on liquid diets than women —at first—because they more often couple their eating program with exercise and because they are often on a liquid diet because of a doctor's strict orders to reduce their weight.

But where a woman will follow the program's or a doctor's instructions, a man on a liquid diet will treat it like he would a project at work; if the goal is to lose 10 pounds in two months by drinking two shakes and eating one solid meal a day, then he'll show everybody how successful a dieter he is by drinking three shakes a day, eating *no* meals, and losing 30 pounds.

Result? If he doesn't cause himself kidney and gallstone trouble by starving himself, he will lose significant muscle tissue as the body burns anything with protein in it to keep on functioning. And since *efficient* weight loss relies on the presence of adequate muscle tissue to burn fat, loss of body fat will be slowed. Muscle loss is what gives men who've lost weight too rapidly that sunken, half-starved look.

Bored with not having something to sink his teeth into, the liquid-fed man will suddenly go back to his old eating habits. The only difference: now he'll keep on drinking the diet shakes to try and convince himself that he's still doing something about his weight.

MEN AND DIET PLATEAUS

This is one weight-related area where men and women have something in common: once he does get onto some kind of weight-loss program, a man is just as likely as a woman to run into a diet plateau (a period where weight loss seemingly stops, and the dieter often gets depressed) after a period of rapid initial loss.

The physiological reasons for leveling off are the same in men and women, too. Much of the loss in the first days of a diet is water. Then the body will grow accustomed to the reduced number of calories coming in and will burn fat more slowly to compensate—even if you're exercising. And a third reason is that even after you or your man have burned the fat from a fat cell, both your bodies will replace it with salty water, which has density and weight, for a few days. Then the cell will gradually empty itself. And both sexes very often "plateau" because they've really started eating wrong again, and they're just trying to deny it. In fact, one of the rare couples who came to me to lose complained that neither of them had lost a pound after they'd made it halfway to their desired weight. They were sure that Mother Nature had it in for them. So I asked them to write down *exactly* what they ate for the next three days. Sure enough, twice a day things like "one pack Ho-Ho's" and "Two rolls with butter" popped up. They were actually rewarding each other for having done so well—and holding up the rest of the show in the meantime.

But for the average man, one of the most important keys to his weight problems that you have probably noticed lies in the late afternoon. And it involves sugar.

MEN AND SUGAR

One of the first things I realized when I started to treat over-weight men was that they have a real problem with sugar, one that very few women suffer from. John Simmons's story is a pretty typical one for the men under my care.

Cutting down on the food at regular meal times was one thing, but it'd get to be about four o'clock in the afternoon and I'd go crazy for something sweet—it was worse than trying to give up the booze, which I'd done about three years ago. I'd actually get faint if I didn't have a candy bar or something. And that'd make me so hungry I had to go down to the taco stand at the corner a couple of hours later.

About 80 percent of obese men (remember, he doesn't have to *look* that big to be obese—a 6-foot man can be unhealthfully overweight at 195 pounds) have a condition called *reactive hypoglycemia*, a stubborn type of low blood sugar that makes bad eating habits particularly hard to break. Women rarely get the condition and men are rarely aware they have it. You're usually left wondering why you find bags of cheap candy all over the house and why he's got to have that bowl of ice cream before he goes to bed. The sugar also makes him fall into a strange, stuporlike sleep at odd times (doctors sometimes call this the "Fat Joe Syndrome"). In fact, many sleep disturbances in men—snoring is one—are caused by too much fat.

The sugar blues for men don't end there. Overweight men with a serious sweet tooth also tend to have a serious lack of *serotonin*, a substance produced by the brain that helps give us our feeling of health and well-being. You've probably noticed he sometimes suffers from depression—lack of interest in you and everybody else around him and deep feelings of self-doubt. A shortage of serotonin and too much sugar can be the cause.

WHY ARE MEN WEIGHT-IGNORANT?

Men gain weight, cope with weight, and suffer because of weight in far different ways than do you. But my twenty years of experience treating women with weight problems has taught me that women have a far better understanding of weight problems than men and are far more likely to take action to correct the problem and move forward. Men are simply blind to the possibility that their beer belly is causing them to look lousy to the women in their life, that it's holding them back in their careers, and in the end, killing them before their time. Here are some of the ways men pay for their weight, according to George Bray, M.D., nationally recognized obesity authority from UCLA and author of *Diet and Obesity* (Saunders, 1989):

- Twenty percent of high blood pressure cases among men are due to flab—and high blood pressure kills 500,000 men every year.
- Eighty percent of type-2 diabetes in men (it can result in blindness and gangrene) is caused by fat.
- Obese men are *three times* more likely than normal men to have high cholesterol levels and heart disease.
- Men who are just 20 percent above their ideal body weight are *five times* more likely than normal-weight men to die before age fifty from an obesity-related disease.

The only person who can really get through to a man about his weight is *you*, the woman in his life. A doctor's warning may help, but by then the damage is usually done—it's a little like calling the fireman after the house has burned down.

You can help educate him, help him gradually learn to eat what's right all the time—in short, help him maintain his body in the best condition possible. And the process can provide emotional cement to a relationship that's been cracking under the strain of too many pounds. Larry Strandberg was a patient of mine with diabetes whose wife, Joy, finally asked me how to deal with his habits. She was afraid she'd lose him. After he'd shed 80 pounds with her help, and *most important*, had kept it off for two years, he finally admitted:

> She was a saint about the whole thing. She didn't nag me, but she did help me out, even though I must have been a pain in the ass. We learned to work together to improve what we had when we first met, and it's gone beyond just eating. It's really changed the kind of relationship we have. For the better.

Your man being overweight has probably caused you more personal unhappiness than you realize, since overeating is often symptomatic of deeper personal problems that extend beyond the refrigerator door. It can, however, cause you even more unnecessary trouble if you let the situation deteriorate. Your man's over-weight is not just another problem that you're supposed to "solve"—it's an area where you are in a unique position to help someone who matters to you—and to help yourself—when no one else can. It's like being the only doctor on an airborne plane when someone keels over; you drop what you're doing and lend a hand, fast. But to do him any real good, to fully comprehend the man's attitude toward his own weight and toward you, you have to go back into his past and understand that problems with the man begin with the boy.

CHAPTER TWO

Boys Are Husky, Girls Are Chubby: How Men Are Brought Up To Eat Too Much

At about seventeen, long before I really started to blow up like a Butterball turkey when I was in my thirties, a friend of mine and I were sitting out in the backyard of my father's place south of Belle-vue, Kentucky. We were doing what boys that age do so well: bragging, about anything and everything. Each of us was trying to go the other one better at sports, girls—and food. When the competition got really fierce (he claimed to have eaten twenty-two blueberry pancakes the previous meal), I turned to the bushel basket of corn up on the porch and said, "Dwayne, I'll go you ear for ear to see who can get to the bottom of that basket first."

One hour and eighteen ears of corn later, I'd won the battle—but lost the war. My future wife held my head while my need to prove my manhood left me sick as a dog. And I'd have done it again in a minute—as long as it was Diana and not Dwayne who saw me turning green in that roadside ditch. Now, I wasn't *born* thinking it was okay to eat myself into a stupor but not okay to be sick in front of another male, but by the time I was seventeen, that assumption seemed to be as much a part of me as my eye color—and it would cause me a lot more trouble in years to come.

THE ROOTS OF MEN'S FAT

In the past couple of years, there's been a lot of noise in the medical community about whether your weight is something predetermined by your genes, which you can't do anything about, or whether your weight will respond to changes in behavior. I feel this is a dangerous trend; science aside, it's like telling people to give up before they've even taken a shot at bettering themselves—and that goes for many situations besides weight loss.

Yes, it is true that genetics has a powerful influence on weight gain, among men as well as women. William E. Dietz, M.D., Chief of Nutrition of the New England Medical Centers in Boston, conducted a study not too long ago which showed that a man with two thin parents has only a 14 percent likelihood of becoming obese at any point in his adult life, while a man with *both* an overweight mother and father has an 80 to 85 percent chance of ending up at the wrong end of the scale. But then comes the wrench in the works: Dr. Dietz also found that if a boy with two thin parents has an obese *baby-sitter* for any substantial period of time, there's a 65 percent chance that he'll become an overweight adult. Conclusion? Socialization factors—how a boy learns to look at food from the example and instruction of his elders—is at least as important as genetics when it comes to men and weight gain.

LIKE FATHER, LIKE SON

Boys naturally turn to their fathers as role models in their early years. They imitate every aspect of their dad's behavior—including what he does at the table, his appearance, and what he believes the male role to be. George Mahan, a banker who was forty-two years old and just as many pounds overweight when he came to me, is typical of how many men related to their father at the dinner table.

My dad owned a small department store and always seemed too busy to spend a lot of time with me. He was bigger than life

to a skinny eight-year-old. Later, I realized he was just *too* big, physically—he died of a heart attack when he was fifty-eight. Anyway, he used to lean over during dinner and tap on my plate if I'd left anything on it. That was a signal for me to eat it all—or else—even if I was stuffed. And it's not like the portions were designed for a kid, either.

I got George to lose weight by cutting down on his portion sizes, and by changing some of his high-fat regular foods to low-fat substitutes that didn't seem too different from the "real" thing. But it took over a year, and the hardest habit to break was his tendency of overfill his plate at every meal, while he was groaning about being full. And even though it was his father who'd make him take out the garbage for a week if he didn't gobble everything down, it was his mother who cooked and spooned out his portion size.

MOTHERS AND SONS

As I've already pointed out, the majority of men who develop a weight problem as post-thirty adults were not obese as boys. Nonetheless, the roots of bad eating habits were being put down during those years, and mothers played a significant if well-intentioned role in the planting.

Despite the fact that the boy wanted to emulate his father, Dad was often a distant character who appeared around dinnertime and then disappeared into television or radio, the paper, work brought home, and then a loud snore. The real emotional connection was with his mother, and that tie was often bound by food.

Henry Robinson, a weight-loss patient of mine, told me his boyhood daily routine, and I find it reflects how a lot of men who are now in their mid-thirties and older learned to relate to their mothers and to food.

The best times I had with my mom were at lunch, when I'd come in from school and she'd have my meal waiting for me.

Those were some of our nicest times, talking together over a meal without the pressure of having my father or anybody else around to interfere.

What Henry experienced was something I've seen many times: a parent using food as a means of showing affection. Even though women are generally better equipped to express themselves emotionally than men, sharing food with male children is a not uncommon way for mothers to express love for their sons. Many women, especially a generation or two ago, wanted to show their sons some affection, but were prevented by the belief that emotional displays could "weaken" a male child. Fixing a plate of pancakes and sausage or a pork sandwich was the only way many women had of saying "I love you" to their sons.

It would be one thing if the food being fixed was good for the boy, but many moms who stopped their sons from snacking between meals, eating too many donuts or bags of candy thought nothing of slathering mayonnaise on a fatty bologna sandwich. Twenty, thirty, or even ten years ago, there wasn't the information available we have today about the role of fat in weight gain and about what you can do to keep fat out of your and your children's diets. What was thought of as good, solid All-American food wasn't known to be the good-tasting but gut-busting wolf in sheep's clothing we know today. Also, the food industry was in an infantile state, with virtually *none* of the low-fat, leaner meats, substitute dairy products, or sweeteners we have today. The worst thing that moms of the '50s and '60s did was believe what they were told. The result? A nation populated with too many men who reach their adult years with a skewered idea of what proper eating, healthy foods, and reasonable portions are all about.

As for boys needing extra fat or having more of a sweet tooth because they're growing, that's hogwash. For certain medical conditions, boys may have some specific nutritional needs, but I can't think of a single case where that means eating more; it means eating more wisely.

Although Mom may have stopped her boy from eating too much, in most homes limits on the young male appetite were usually set *only* if the boy was obviously overweight; otherwise, boys were encouraged to eat and eat and eat—well beyond their natural inclination. Very early on, eating was equated with size, and size was equated with masculinity, a belief that causes plenty of trouble when the same boy grows up to be a sedentary man. How many men can recall, if you give them a chance, being almost force-fed as boys? Harold Conrad, who came to me at age thirty-seven with 75 excess pounds and a nascent case of noninsulin diabetes, recalls his boyhood eating habits.

> I didn't get heavy until I was about thirty. As a kid and teen-ager I was a pretty normal weight. But I did get into the habit of stuffing myself when and where I pleased. In fact, my mother and everybody else were always telling me things like "Clean your plate so you can have dessert," or, "You're a boy; you need to eat or you'll get sick," so I ended up with a bad habit of eating everything in sight, even when I wasn't hungry. Funny, though—my parents were always telling my younger sister to stop eating like a pig or she'd never make cheerleader, even when she was just picking at her plate. She ended up so self-conscious about food that she'd eat practically nothing at mealtime. She'd just sit there and stare at her plate.

STUFF A SON, STARVE A DAUGHTER

Harold's recollections present a typical picture of the American table a few years ago, and, unfortunately, things have not changed all that much. My observation is that, pretty consistently, boys were and are taught to eat too much and girls pressured to eat too little. Thus is created an unhealthy situation where women come of age with an unnatural self-consciousness about food—a tendency to snack obsessively on the sly while skimping at main meals. Girls were and are taught to view food as an enemy or adversary and eating as something to be ashamed of. Or worse, some young girls blame food for a body that doesn't fit the popular image of perfection, and develop life-threatening eating disorders such as anorexia or bulimia. They become so self-conscious about food they're caught in a binge and purge cycle or they won't eat at all. Both conditions are extremely dangerous, and they're a result not of any natural vulnerability on the part of women (as in the case with breast cancer or osteoporosis) but of *conditioning* by parents and society. The same is true of boys, and although as men they don't suffer from the same eating disorders that women become trapped by, they are still headed toward ill health, ignorant of the roots of their problem—or still unable and unwilling to admit that they have any problem at all.

STATUS AND SIZE

Although I've found that there is a correlation between weight conscious and economic status (the higher the family income, the more attention paid to keeping children's weight within healthful limits), that wasn't true years ago—there was no knowledge for educated people to act on—and I've discovered that men in higher-status jobs equate size and masculinity just as often as their blue-collar counterparts, as a direct result of their experiences as a youth. One major auto industry captain I know of, very highly placed, was banished to a fitness spa by his doctor and was brought down from a bursting at the seams 220 to a trim 165 pounds. He told his doctor when he left, though, that he wasn't afraid of gaining the weight back—he was afraid his younger subordinates would view him as "a skinny guy they can step on, just like when I was a kid."

TV AND HIS INNER TUBE

Mom, Dad, and the situation at home were not the only sources of your man's present weight woes; our national addiction to television has contributed to the image of men as big eaters who

gorge themselves without any consequences. The situation come-
dies of the '50s and '60s were especially guilty of promoting male
overeating. Women were always shown preparing food (and their
helpers were always daughters, not sons). Who doesn't remember
"My Three Sons"? In the kitchen scenes, Robbie, Chip, and Ernie
were always swinging open the fridge door for something to eat—
like a triple-decker sandwich or something similar.

Even later when you had relatively sophisticated shows such as
"All in the Family," the same basic attitudes toward male and female
consumption of food were promoted: Meathead's piglike eating habits may have been ridiculed (never by women, only by Archie), but
you never saw Gloria or Edith permitted the same relationship to
food. Again, the casual—and especially the young—viewer was left
with the impression that men eat what they want when they want to.
The overall impression was that positive female role models didn't eat
anything at all. They only cooked and bought groceries.

Have things changed much over the past twenty years? Not
really. If you take a look at most current television shows, men are
still shown gorging and women picking. "Roseanne" is a step forward, in that Roseanne Arnold ridicules her husband for his overweight almost as much as he makes fun of her. Whenever I watch
that show I just want to yell at the set and tell both of them to drop
a few pounds if they want to live to see their grandchildren graduate
from high school. What makes me especially mad is that they don't
even think seriously about their weight—which is a pretty good sign
that their children and grandchildren won't either.

SELLING THE OVERWEIGHT MAN

The advertising industry hasn't been of much help in the wors-
ening of our national male weight problem, either. Men have always been depicted in advertisements as bottomless pits for high-fat
foods, beer, and every kind of gut-busting snack the ad men could
dream up. I remember one that particularly bothered me, from the
Bob's Big Boy chain (think about that name) when it opened in the

South during the 1950s. The billboard ad had a picture of a big, sloppy guy for its come-on. It showed him stuffing an oversized burger covered with cheese and every other heart attack–promoting topping into his mouth, with what looked like a barrel of beer sitting in a glass next to him, waiting to join the party around his waist. What did the eight- or ten-year-old boy driving by make of that? I'll tell you: He took it as yet another message that this was how grown-up men were supposed to eat and look. And I'll guarantee you that he *does* look at least a little like that thirty years later. As a now forty-year-old male patient of mine remembers, "When I was growing up, bigger was always considered better if you were a boy. Everything around us, TV, our parents, told us that. Not eating a lot was kind of—well, *girls* weren't supposed to eat a lot. Nobody told us about the heart attack stuff, though."

It's only in recent years—perhaps the last two, at most—that some of the liquid diet programs have used men in their advertisements (what they don't tell them is that 90 to 95 percent of men will gain back the weight they lose on these fasts within twenty-four months, just like women). And that's too late for the boys who became men thinking it was not only right, but their duty, to eat themselves into an early grave.

BOYS IN THE LOCKER ROOM

Once a boy is beyond the age of ten or so, his ideas about eating and size are shaped as much by his experiences outside the home as within it. While he may have a couple of crude classes on nutrition in school (probably on eating from the "four food groups" and how to brush his teeth: "down on the uppers and up on the lowers"), the most powerful influence will come from the athletics department in his school.

Athletic teams and gym classes have, aside from some positive things (like a basic sense of what exercise is) fostered misconceptions among young men about healthy weight. I can't tell you how many times fathers have brought their eleven-, twelve-, or sixteen-year-old boys into me, not to help them *lose* weight, but to *gain* it—even if they are a perfectly normal weight. Dad is usually 20 or 30 pounds the wrong side of the scale himself. Often, he'll want his boy to go well over the recommended weight for his age in order to make a sports team—either a sport that Dad played himself or one that he wanted to. It's usually football.

The coaches go along with this; their jobs are dependent on their teams' winning and, especially in football, the big guy wins. So they end up sentencing these young boys to years or possibly a lifetime of bad eating habits to fulfill their own goals. The boy becomes confused. Even though he may feel physically uncomfortable with the weight squeezing in on him, he learns that there are rewards to being "husky" (read *fat*) that are important to him, and will remain important to him as a grown man. He has the approval of his peers, his parents, and the whole adult world. He feels that, even if he's not entirely comfortable with it, his extra weight offers both protection and power, and that he has to keep eating in order to maintain a sense of his own masculinity. Again, as I pointed out in the last chapter, I'm not talking about obviously fat boys, who are in the minority. I'm talking about the kid who is simply too big for his height *and* I'm talking about all the other boys who stuff themselves because they want to be just like him.

As an adult, this same boy may manage to keep his physique and his health through his twenties. He might continue to keep up some sort of physical activity, or he might just be lucky enough to have a genetic heritage that lets him stave off the inevitable for a few years. But when he hits thirty, the natural slowdown of his metabolism will result in the paunch, "love handles," and the beginnings of other, internal physical problems discussed in Chapter 1 that are caused by the overeating he learned as a boy.

Randy Colters was always the "big guy" in school, from grammar school through college. He fulfilled his father's and his own dream by making quarterback on his high school team, then taking the same position at the state university. After rising through an old boys' network to become vice-president of sales for an office supply company before he was forty, Randy found that he'd "gone soft," as he put it to me, and wanted advice on how he could get back into "fighting form." In all too typical fashion, he was afraid that he would be unable to compete with younger, thinner men.

What was required—and it was an especially rough case because Randy was newly separated from his wife and had no one to check his progress on a daily basis—was not getting him to lose weight, but convincing him that his boyhood habit of eating two or three times as much food as his body needed, had to stop. He'd always bring up how much he ate when he played and how he didn't eat any more now than he did twenty years ago, and if his eating habits didn't do him any harm back then, why did they matter now and how come I just couldn't put him on a liquid diet for a few weeks and call it a day?

I told Randy what I tell everyone who comes up with that question: Now, it's true that *if* a grown man kept up his boyhood gobbling habits *and* exercised vigorously (with a combination weight training and cardiovascular workout) for one to two hours a day, he would have less of a fat appearance and less of a potential for a health problem, but that's just not in the cards for men who have a family, a relationship, or a reasonably demanding job. The road to health would have been a lot easier if he'd been taught as a youngster to eat in moderation and to eat sensible, low-fat foods.

I put my own two boys on a weight-gain diet when they were teen-agers so they could play ball: almost 5,000 calories a day, and an awful lot of them from fat. I made sure that they got the kind of daily workout that they needed to burn the fat off and grow muscle, but to this day I'm sorry I let them talk me into it. There's a happy ending in their case, though. After they graduated from college, they both dropped their calorie intake back to a normal level and, through mixing weight training with cardiovascular exercise, they're at a perfect weight for their age and height. However, I'd never let anyone talk me into doing the same thing again.

FREEING YOUR BOY FROM FUTURE FAT

I'm often asked by mothers today, especially when they've just licked a weight problem themselves, what they can do to prevent their sons from growing up with eating habits and attitudes toward food that'll almost insure they'll be overweight by the time they're forty.

First, if you have an overweight man in the house who makes a public display of his overeating, your task is going to be more difficult. No matter what you do, that man is going to be a role model for the boy, and a bad influence in terms of eating habits. If you're a single parent and assuming your own weight is under control, the job's a little easier.

- Fat-proof your house. Following the food-buying recommendations in Chapter 7, keep all high-fat foods out of your kitchen. Beware the hidden fats in sauces, sandwich condiments, and other seemingly harmless foods.
- Communicate to your son what the health consequences of being overweight are: there's nothing wrong with talking at an early age about the threat that being overweight can pose, especially if the boy is overeating and developing bad eating habits and doesn't have to put up with ridicule because of his weight. That's the kind of boy who has difficulty connecting food causes with physical effects later on. I hate to sound like a schoolmarm, but as is the case with sexually transmitted diseases, forewarned is forearmed.
- Using the recommendations in Chapter 7 as a guide, encourage your son to eat reasonable portions at mealtime, and don't let him overeat. Encourage *both* your girls and your boys to observe the same moderate, low-fat eating habits. Be on guard against encouraging a double standard in eating habits between boys and girls.
- Let your son know that eating is not a game and not a competition—there are many other ways for him to prove himself than on a dinner plate.
- Establish sensible eating habits in boys *and* girls before they enter their teen years. Bad eating patterns, like most other things, are difficult to break once age thirteen comes around.
- Don't stuff your boy. If he says he's through with his meal and he's had a reasonable variety of foods, don't insist that he eat more—he'll begin to associate overeating with your approval.
- If your kids are going to eat fast food, make sure they know what the low-fat choices on the fast-food menus are; most of the big

chains like McDonald's have at least one acceptable item these days.

Remember that you can exercise great influence over how your son (or daughter) will view food as an adult. Use that power before a difficult job becomes next to impossible, and your child pays the price.

WHEN THE BOY BECOMES A MAN

There's nothing you can do to change the way the overweight man in your life was raised, but knowing where he's coming from, at least as far as attitude toward food, will help you understand why it's so difficult for him to even *conceive* of having a weight problem. Here, as in so many things, there's failure in male/female communication. You look at the problem from the point of view of someone who was raised to think of overweight too *much*, and he looks at it from the point of someone who was taught to think of it too *little*. So what do you end up with? A man who looks in the mirror and sees O. J. Simpson when you're thinking more along the lines of John Candy.

CHAPTER THREE

The Quarterback
in the Mirror:
What He Sees
When You See Fat

Think back for a minute on the last high school or college reunion you went to and how concerned you were about your appearance. Most adult women I know make a conscious appraisal about whether they should lose a few pounds during the weeks before an event like this. It doesn't have to be a reunion, either. It could be a wedding, a bar mitzvah, a christening—any event where you're going to run into people who haven't seen you for a long time.

Not so with men. I'll bet when you got to that reunion and looked around at the guys (especially the former jocks), you found that a lot of them seemed to have changed *substantially*, appearance-wise—and not for the better. The captain of the football team, the school stud ten or twenty years before, probably looked like he was wearing a Jello-O mold around his waist. But then—this is the kicker—so did the gawky, skinny guy who used to stuff himself with cafeteria Sloppy Joes hoping to put some meat on his bones.

We've already taken a look at the food/eating value system men develop as boys: how, unlike girls, they are encouraged to stuff themselves and to eat much more than they need to—and all this with high-fat foods that would give a heart attack to a bull elephant. It is not surprising, therefore, that they take this attitude with them as they gorge their way toward manhood.

47

From teen-age years through young adulthood, men engrave their overeating patterns in stone. As we've seen, because of their metabolism and because (again, unlike women) neither their burgeoning size nor their eating habits are subjected to the criticism of society, they reach age thirty without any concept of what *fat* really means.

To overweight adult men, fat is a feminine word and dieting is a feminine activity. In other words, fat is a "weakness." They're scared to death that somehow they'll be less of a man if they look in the mirror and say to themselves, "George, you need to lose some *fat*"—or if anyone says it to them. When their post-thirty day of reckoning comes, they find it impossible to use the F-word in reference to themselves, either when talking to others (including their doctors) or when they look at themselves in the mirror.

WHAT THE FAT MAN SEES

When dealing with the overweight men who come to me of their own accord or in tandem with their wives, I have to approach them on a whole different level than I would you. These men, who just by virtue of being in my waiting room are much more aware of the health problems associated with too much fat than are other males, won't admit that they have too much weight on their bodies. They have a vocabulary all their own, and one that women are usually unaware of. To women, *fat* is *fat* and that's that. But men not only have a spare tire between them and good health, they also have a language problem when it comes to honest self-description:

"I'm getting a little bit *soft*, Doc."

"Geez, if only I had time to work out like I used to, I could get this *muscle toned*."

"I don't know what it is, Dr. Sutkamp, but I'm really *getting out of shape*."

Did you notice that the words *fat* and *overweight* and *I eat too much* are nowhere to be found? It's hard to believe, but I even had a difficult time getting men who are already beset by weight-related physical problems such as diabetes and cardiovascular disease to use the word *fat* when they talk about their own condition and the reasons for it. This is true of men from all classes; single, married, or divorced; black or white; bald or with a full head of hair.

So what do they think they're in my office for? Well, they've usually found out that their blood pressure is up, that they have high cholesterol, an irregular heartbeat, a sugar imbalance or some other physical problem caused by the extra 30 to 40 pounds they've been carrying around (as mentioned earlier, most overweight, post-thirty men are about that much the wrong side of the scale). Most try to get me (as I'm sure they do you) to participate in their denial games by simply writing them a prescription and telling them they need to exercise a little bit—which they have no intention of doing anyway.

EILEEN ERICKSON

My son, Harry, was just thirty-one and living at home after his divorce. His wife got the house and even though he could afford it, I think he liked having me cook and do his laundry for him. His career was in great shape—he was the classic up-and-coming young lawyer—but he was used to that kind of success, since he'd been the captain of every sports team in high school and college. But his job meant he was eating too much and not getting any exercise, and he started looking just like his father did at his age—puffy, the star player gone to seed. He would never say that he'd gained too much weight—he'd just insist he needed to get "back to the track," or "go to the gym again"—that sort of thing. But he didn't do a thing about it and the quarts of Häagen-Dazs just kept on going from the freezer right into his mouth and onto his waist.

IS HIS FLAB REALLY JUST "SOFT MUSCLE"?

Before we talk any more about the self-perception of the overweight man and how it affects your life with him, let's dispense with a couple of common questions concerning the physical facts about the adult male. That way, whether you say anything or not, you won't have to ask yourself whether *you're* the crazy one the next time he starts throwing the bull around.

Q. Can "flaccid" muscle cause me to look overweight? Can male muscle "turn to fat?"
A. No, plain and simple. Inactivity may contribute to a generally unhealthy appearance in a man, but unused muscles don't drop down around his waist and they don't get bigger with more beer and donuts. The old myth about muscle turning to fat is just a load of bull he uses to kid himself. Fat is fat and muscle is muscle and that's the bottom line.

Q. Can muscle toning exercise—like weight lifting—alone rid a man of overweight?
A. No. He might enjoy a slightly improved appearance through exercise by toning the muscle which is underneath the fat (the same is true of women, though your muscles tend to be smaller and you won't get as dramatic a result from weight training), but he won't be getting rid of any substantial amount of fat unless and until he changes his eating habits. If he does start doing a little bit of exercise, it's usually to pump his biceps and upper chest; that's why you'll see so many "fit" men with muscular arms and a big gut down below. That doesn't do him any good at all. And the way the pattern usually works with men, he'll probably take doing any sort of exercise as a license to eat even more fatty foods.

THE MALE STATE OF DENIAL

The average man's perspective with regard to his own overweight is very similar to that of an unrepentant drug user or alcoholic (although certainly the consequences of the behavior are not as devastating). Overweight men in their thirties, forties, or older have been taught all their life that their way of eating is the right way. As a result, they have an adolescent personality when it comes to the subject of food and how it relates to their own body image. In their minds, the words *big* and *brawny* are the same.

The level of self-deception and denial among these men can be pretty startling, especially for the women they're involved with.

SOPHIE ROLLINS

Bob and I used to go out to dinner at one of the local restaurants once in a while, even though I tried to avoid it because he already had a 42-inch waist. We were living down South at the time and he'd order ribs, biscuits, and gravy—you name it and it was on his plate and in his belly before you could blink. Then he'd lean back and say, "Honey, do you really think you *should?*" if I had so much as a dish of rice pudding. It got so bad that I finally lost my temper one day and pointed right across the table at his middle and said, "I am *not* the fat one in this family." It didn't do any good though. He had to get diabetes before he'd listen to the doctor and change how he ate.

SUCCESSFUL LOSERS

Strangely enough, the only men I've met who will initiate their own weight-reduction program are the ones I spoke about in the last chapter: the gynoid men who were overweight themselves as boys or adolescents, with most of their fat on the lower half of the body. They tend to have a perspective on weight in common with women in that they think they need to lose more weight than they really do. When they come to me, they'll think they have 30 or 40 pounds to lose when they really have only 20.

Jimmy Nachman was a pretty typical case. He'd been a bell-shaped overeater since age ten, with the kind of fine, almost hairless skin that men with the gynoid body type often have. He first came to me when he was twenty-two years old, just under 6 feet tall but with almost 300 pounds packed onto his frame, determined to rid himself of the fat that had caused him such a painful adolescence. He not only changed his eating habits, he also became an avid, almost obsessive runner. He did lose well over 100 pounds, but he would come back to my office even if he picked up 5 extra pounds over the holidays, in a panic and thinking he'd put on a ton.

JIMMY NACHAM

If I look in the mirror and see even a little bit of extra weight, or if the scale at my health club shows even a couple of pounds more than the week before, I go crazy to lose it. All I can think of is being a fat boy again and all the pain I went through because of it. Never again.

It's all a matter of what kind of eating philosophy and physical self-image you acquire at an early age. These men are scared to death that they're going to go back to being the one everybody made fun of—the pudgy kid who couldn't get a date and was always picked last when sides were chosen for gym-class teams. Even though these men will probably never have the classic, V-shaped male physique that others have, they're much better at maintaining their health once they get into their thirties. Unfortunately, they're the exception among men, not the rule.

IN HIS MIND, SIZE EQUALS SUCCESS

It's not just the former King of the Hop who buys into the bigger-is-better syndrome. The skinny guy who used to get sand kicked in his face affects it as well. *Size* was always something these now large individuals pursued by eating, eating, eating throughout their high school and college years because they thought it was the key to male happiness.

GEORGE OLIN

When I was in college, I used to eat *five* meals a day—not the nutritious stuff, either, but any kind of garbage from the vending machines in the school library. It was 6 foot 2 inches and weighed 145 pounds. Talk about Ichabod Crane! I used to wear long underwear in June just to make myself look heavier. I wanted to be like the big guys—you know, the ones who got the girls, the scholarships, all that. But by the time I started putting on the weight I'd always wanted, I was in my early thirties, and it was the wrong kind. I guess I still must believe in that image, too, even though I lost the weight a couple of years ago because of my health. Even though I know being heavy is bad for my health, I'm still just not comfortable, mentally at least, with being skinny.

George and most other men who were thin when they were young reach adulthood with a skewed idea of what *skinny* actually means. Because of the mythology that surrounds the idea of being *big* for teenage boys, they reach full manhood and middle age thinking *smaller* means *lesser*. Size is associated with privilege, eating voraciously with taking one's due. It gets to be a habit, and the belief carries through to the whole value system that males are taught, across the board. All you need to do is look around him to see why he's blind to his own weight. Although we American men are changing, we still tend to believe that bigger houses, bigger cars, bigger meals—everything we own or are has to be *oversize* to reinforce a healthy sense of our own masculinity. And anything that threatens that masculinity is at first rejected, even if it involves preserving health. That is, until he's facing a do-or-die situation.

MAN AS BREADWINNER, MAN AS DOUGHBOY

Along with these perceptions carried over from his youth, the "big guy" often feels, deep down, that he *deserves* to eat massive quantities of food because he is the mainstay of the family income. This, even though an army of social scientists (as well as a separate battalion of working women) can tell him that it just ain't so anymore.

JACK PIURKOWSKI
When I was still over 250 pounds, I'd get home at night and be worn out from dealing with customers all day. I felt like food

was a reward for my working so hard. I felt that I deserved to eat like some guys feel they deserve a Scotch or a beer. And even though my wife was putting in a full day selling real estate, I felt more comfortable pigging out than she did. Looking back, I can see a lot of my father in me, that way.

MEN, WEIGHT, AND WORK

Work and work-related circumstances such as having to travel a lot, often provide men with what seem to them logical reasons for puffing up to gargantuan proportions. They don't look at these as excuses, as such, but rather from the perspective of, "Well, this is what it is to be a *man*." It's all part of a general pattern of self-deception about what they look like and how they got that way. Some of the more common claims:

"The food on the plane is awful, but I've got to eat it."

"In my business, I've got to eat out a lot."

"I can't let my client/customer eat alone."

"These guys expect you to drink with them—if you don't, the other guy gets the business."

"There's no way I can lose weight while I've got this job—it goes with the territory."

STRESS AND MALE OVEREATING

There is another side to the coin. You have to understand that, whatever they say and however much macho swagger is in their attitude about eating, many overweight men are at an uncomfortable spot on the scale because of underlying stress. As with alcohol, food is often used, subconsciously or not, as a form of medication. Along with their long-ingrained belief that overeating is a male birthright, men use food, like cigarettes and an after-work cocktail or beer, to calm themselves in the face of a hostile world which they've decided they have to take on alone.

A few years ago I had a male patient, Dave Bulliam, who had come to me because he'd finally developed obesity-related diabetes at age forty-three after ballooning up to 310 pounds several years earlier. I had to put him on a liquid diet for a short period, which I hate doing. But it was the only way to reduce the immediate threat to his life and to prevent further deterioration of his condition.

He lost a great deal of weight back then, but six months ago he walked back into my office looking, if anything, worse than before. "Dave!" I said. "What the hell happened to you? You're not only off the wagon, you're in the ditch on the side of a dirt road!"

Dave was a blue-collar kind of guy who'd made good at a tire distribution company that he now owned. He went into a long tale of lawsuits, counter-lawsuits, arrests for graft, in-laws who stole money from him—a regular "Dallas."

The difference was that he seemed to think that eating was a logical accompaniment to his troubles, like ketchup with French fries. There was real regret on his part because his health was affected, but he didn't seem to feel this was a logical consequence of his behavior. He just thought it was unfair that a man with his responsibilities should be prevented from eating.

COMMUNICATING ABOUT WEIGHT

Most women cannot comprehend how men can look at themselves and not see the obvious: *fat*. As an American woman of any age, you arrive at your adult destination with years of weight training, sometimes seeing extra pounds where there may be none. Many women, and the rare man like Jimmy Nacham, verge on being overly concerned about potential overweight. That attitude comes from spending your formative years badgered by parents, teachers, and peers who insisted that, just as bigger is better for boys, thin is in for girls.

Despite the tremendous problem Americans have with changing our fatty diets, and the number of overweight people in this country, the emphasis on being thin for women has often had young girls ruining their eating patterns at a very young age in pursuit of an "ideal" weight that they'll never reach. Boys do the same thing, but at the opposite end of the spectrum. As a result, we have an entire generation (or two) of men and women who can't communicate about *weight*.

WENDY AND BILL HOCHSTED

Wendy Hochsted was at a perfectly normal weight herself—she'd sometimes go a little bit above her so-called ideal weight, but nothing serious. She made an appointment with me one day to discuss, not *her* weight, but her husband Bill's problem. He was getting bigger, as she put it, "by the minute." He'd just turned thirty-nine, was an educated, professional man, but he seemed totally unconcerned about his expanding girth. With a history of heart disease and early death among the males in his family, she was worried about him.

Bill was rising faster and faster on the career ladder, and the higher his position became, the more weight he seemed to gain. Wendy swore that "for every extra $10,000 he earns, he brings home an extra 10 pounds with it." She was unhappy with him on a variety of levels (she didn't come right out and say it, but I gather he wasn't a pretty sight when the bathrobe came off at night), and she couldn't understand his total lack of concern about his weight and health. He would cheerfully go out and buy a new set of expensive clothes twice a year to hold his expanding girth (I call this style of dressing "sausage casing") and made a habit of celebrating each new success with a night out in an expensive restaurant.

At first, Wendy took the silent-sufferer tack, thinking that the situation would right itself; after all, Bill was an intelligent guy in all other respects. She was sure he'd lose on his own. He didn't. Then she got angry and took a more aggressive course. She criticized the way he looked, began to ridicule him, calling him fat, then a fat load and slob, and capped it off by refusing to accompany him on any of his feeding frenzies. Here's how one of their fat fights would start.

> WENDY: (Eying him tensely as he ladels himself a bowl of ice cream at 11:00 P.M.) You know, my mother was just saying the other day she couldn't believe the man I'd married had gotten to look so much like Dom DeLuise.
>
> BILL: Well, did you tell her that Dom DeLuise was paying for the plate of food in front of her? If I'm Dom DeLuise, she's Roseanne's grandmother.

This kind of conversation consists of two people talking *at*, not *with* each other. These two intelligent people ended up not communicating on any level—all because of 70 or 80 pounds of greasy fat globules wrapped around his chest.

Wendy and Bill have reached a weight communications impasse. Each has an entirely different perception of the situation. He believes she is trying to emasculate him with criticism of his weight at a time when he feels he's proving his mettle as a man with financial success. In his mind, by attacking his weight, she's attacking his masculinity. She believes that he is displaying reckless disregard for her by both ignoring her genuine concern, her feelings about how she wants her life partner to look, and by his seeming indifference to placing his own health (and therefore their relationship) in mortal danger.

FAT AND THE FRAT MENTALITY

One thing I've noticed that is typical of an overweight man who has a woman in his life bothering him about his weight is that he'll not only give her an angry response or the silent treatment, he'll retreat to the company of his male friends. With them, weight is never the subject (again, men *never* talk about weight amongst themselves) and he can have almost unrestricted access to food with the tacit approval of his peers.

Millie Fenner first noticed her live-in boyfriend's new pattern after she started her campaign against the roll around his middle, acquired during the three years they'd lived together.

MILLIE FENNER

I guess I started nagging a little bit, and then I tried to replace the food he was used to—the steaks and fries and all of that—with healthy, almost vegetarian stuff. Suddenly he dug up all these friends he hadn't seen in years and started telling me he'd be home late from work. From the size of him, they sure weren't out jogging together.

WHAT'S A WOMAN TO DO?

Most women who have overweight men in their house or their lives are silent for too long. Then their anger leads them to explode in ways that are counterproductive to their goal: to have a healthy man of reasonable weight. Here are some tips on how the male mindset works, and how to deal with it.

- From the get-go, assume he doesn't know the meaning of the word *fat*—at least in relation to himself. Try to use his language when you're talking about his overweight, but couple it with the knowledge that you have of dieting and men as a result of reading this book. Examples:

  WON'T WORK: You're getting fat as a hog.

  WILL WORK: You're working too hard and getting a little out of shape.

  WON'T WORK: Do you have to stuff yourself like that?

  WILL WORK: Don't eat so fast! We can't afford to have you sick.

- The real key in communicating about food with a man who has a sense of masculinity tied directly to his food attitudes is not to show aggressiveness or anger. Deep down, overweight men know something is amiss (even if they're just physically uncomfortable from all their extra weight), but they will stay fat rather than sacrifice any part of their male pride.

- Avoid confrontations that make him more stubborn (and probably fatter).
- Persuade him to eat normal amounts of food.
- Help him identify the real reasons and fears for his overeating and how else he might cope with them.
- By informing without insulting, get him to see a true reflection in the mirror—instead of seeing what he wants to see.

CHAPTER FOUR

Your Role in Your Man's Weight Loss

Now that you know how the man in your life sees fat, from birth to adulthood, you're probably wondering—with good cause—what you can possibly do to change his attitude and approach. Since men can be so completely stubborn in changing their habits regarding anything, including food, it might seem next to impossible to get them to look at alternatives, but that's just not so.

Often a woman who tries to interest her man in his own health uses the wrong approach. She'll confront him, not with the facts, but with anger and hostility—and often that anger comes from having waited too long: he's either too overweight or too close to being seriously ill. His response? He will quickly chalk up your genuine concern to histrionics, assume the classic male defense posture of ignoring you and suddenly go completely deaf, where his eating and weight are concerned.

It doesn't have to be that way. You can assume an important role in his weight loss utilizing what you've learned through your own experience and in these pages. Even though women are becoming a more and more significant part of the labor force, they are still, for the most part, in control of the food shopping and food preparation for their households. There's a reason for that: by and large, men are still food, diet and shopping ignorant, for all the reasons discussed in Chapters 1 through 3. This ignorance is one of the things that has to change, even if just a little bit, and you can be the partner who helps him make that change.

HOW MEN HAVE BEEN HANDLED

Back in the nutritional dark ages of the 1960s, '70s and early '80s, women were often advised by a variety of self-appointed experts that the way to handle a man's special nutritional needs was to "trick" him into thinness: just cut down his portion size at dinner, put an apple in his lunch instead of a package of Twinkies and swap the sugar on the table for Nutrasweet—he won't notice. I can tell you here and now that that kind of back-door approach doesn't work with men, and can actually make matters worse. Either that, or male weight problems have been ignored entirely.

CONCHETTA RIOS

When I saw that my son—he was twenty-nine at the time—and my husband were both getting really overweight, I didn't say anything about it, although I was worried. I just stopped buying the things at the store that I felt were bad for them—the pies, the heavy dairy products, the fatty meats, that kind of thing.

It lasted about two weeks. When the two of them weren't complaining that they were "hungry," they'd go out and buy all that garbage food themselves and I'd find it in the refrigerator. Then I realized that at breakfast, after I'd stopped making eggs and bacon and started serving one of those high-fiber cereals, they'd both go *together* to one of those greasy spoons downtown to stuff themselves. So much for the subtle approach.

The "back-door," or trickster approach is doomed to failure when you're dealing with men on both a practical basis—after all, you can't police them for three meals a day—and on a psychological basis. I also find the whole concept of sneaking around someone you're supposed to be close to insulting to both parties.

IS THIS JUST ANOTHER PROBLEM OF HIS I'M EXPECTED TO SOLVE?

Along with all the other burdens women are expected to shoulder (child care, primary domestic responsibility, the pets, the bills and very often holding a full-time job), should their husband's health maintenance be yet another responsibility to take on?

Yes, in some ways. But the practical fact is that you are better informed than he is in this regard. You have been more food-sensitive your entire life, even if you've had weight problems of your own, and you are health-literate enough to have bought this book.

I think it's the responsibility of one human being to impart knowledge that they have to someone who needs it. If you don't, well, that would be as if Dr. Salk held out on giving the public his polio vaccine because he thought people should solve their own problems.

Eventually, your mate *will* take responsibility for himself. My experience is that your man will learn from you if you approach him sensibly and not angrily with what you've learned in this book about the male physiognomy and the male mind. In most cases, after six months of coaching by you, I predict he'll absorb all the good things you've been preaching into his own eating and exercise habits and he'll start to tell you a few things about health and fitness himself.

WHAT WORKS WITH MEN

Men, especially the overweight men who may be in just a little bit of denial about their problem, don't respond well when: 1) as mentioned, someone—man or woman—tries to trick them into doing something; 2) someone tries to get them to do something *without telling them the reason why*.

American males tend to pride themselves on their rationality. They don't like to do anything or make any change in their life just because someone tells them it's good for them. They want to know the cause-and-effect quotient. That's why it's always a good idea to make any problem on which you want him to work a project with a beginning, a middle and an end, something that he can learn. In the case of food and nutrition, you are the educator.

It's not as though you need any more work to do or things to worry about during the course of a day, but the fact is that you are the only person who can effect lasting change in a man's eating habits. I have found over the years that in a *reasonably* healthy relationship (I've yet to see one that's perfect) men respond to women who are *direct* in communicating their knowledge about nutrition and food buying to them. The role of nonjudgmental ally and educator is the most effective part a woman can play in the battle against men's fat.

It's not an easy role to add to the ten or twenty other things a modern woman has to juggle, but it will make a constructive difference to him. Success in helping him change his eating habits can benefit you as well, in ways we'll discuss later in the book.

IS IT JUST HIS WEIGHT?

Before you can begin to extend the knowledge you've gained in these pages and from your own health/diet-related experience, you have to make sure that you're not making your unhappiness with his paunch a proxy for other problems, either in your own life or in your relationship with him. Too often, I've seen a woman focus on her man's eating habits as a source of great frustration to her when, in fact, if he dropped 40 pounds the next day and ate only broiled chicken and high-fiber vegetables for the rest of his life, she'd still be angry with him for something, from making noise while he eats to snoring to leaving the top off of the garbage can to smoking in the house, while avoiding far more basic flaws in the relationship.

MIRIAM STEEGE

After I'd been married for about ten years it seemed like the only conversation I had with Bill was to complain about his eating and weight. God, we got into some knock-down, drag-out battles over it. The argument would always start with how much he was overeating, but it would always move on to something else in short order. I'd hit him on how his clothes didn't fit him anymore, then I'd move on to his bad breath, how he didn't clip his toenails enough—then it would just turn into a free-for-all about how he didn't have any respect for me. I guess that was what our fights were really about. It was just a bad relationship, and my reaction to his weight and his overeating was just a symptom of that fact.

The man's food intake and eating habits very often become the focal point of frustration in a relationship that has many other problems. That's as true from your man's perspective as it is from yours. The problem might be sexual, it might be behavior rooted in his or your childhood that has nothing to do with his eating habits, it can even be a money-related conflict that causes you to quarrel over his weight.

You can recognize nonweight-related conflict that is *expressed* in quarrels that focus on weight by your own reaction. Ask yourself these simple questions:

- Do you feel *anger*, as opposed to concern, toward your man when you discuss or think about his weight and eating habits?
- Do you feel real *anxiety* over his weight when he's in close physical proximity to you?
- Did you have an unhappy relationship with your own overweight father?

If your answer to any one of these three questions is yes, you may want to look deeper to see if there are other conflicts to resolve (preferably in individual therapy or with a marriage counselor) before you can even begin to help your man achieve results with a weight-loss campaign. Otherwise, you'll just be treading water.

How much you can help him also depends on *how* overweight he is—and whether you're overweight yourself. Having a mutual overeating habit isn't that serious a problem if you're both just a few pounds overweight, but if you both are extremely overweight—and getting bigger—then you may be feeding each other's bad habits—

pun intended. That's an eating co-dependency problem, and I always advise patients involved in such a relationship, where food is *too* much of a bond, to seek professional psychological help from support groups, like a local chapter of Overeaters' Anonymous. After that, I tell them, come back to me.

A HELPING HAND

What you must feel when you're dealing with your man is a healthy *concern* for him, not anger. That doesn't mean you can't get *angry* at him, though:

BETTY BRODY

When George started gaining and gaining—he must have been 40 or 50 pounds overweight—I really started to worry. But I didn't know what to do about the situation. We had a terrific marriage, but he just didn't know how to eat. And after he turned thirty, it got to be a very real cause for concern because he naturally started to thicken in the middle. That "gap in his education," as I liked to call it, was putting my terrific marriage in danger. I guess I lost my temper with him a couple of times because I just didn't know how to get him to pay attention to his diet and his eating habits. I guess I was being a little bit selfish about it, but I wanted to keep him around.

YOU'LL BENEFIT, TOO

As a sort of combined teacher/doctor for your man, you'll find that you'll benefit as well from your focus on nutrition and eating, on two levels.

First, you'll begin to accrue the same health benefits that he will if he follows your advice and if he sticks to the meal plan outlined in Chapter 7. My experience with couples has shown that when a woman tries to help her man lose weight, begin to exercise and improve his health, *she* almost inevitably begins to see positive changes in her own habits. It can be anything from losing a few pounds to tightening up your own muscles, or simply making wiser choices in your own eating habits. A woman, I've discovered, may not be as overweight as her man, but she suffers nonetheless from poor nutrition. That's because she is probably, out of habit, eating much the same thing that he is—just not as much of it.

Second, and perhaps more important, you put a welcome dollop of *assertiveness*—not aggressiveness—in your own life when you're dealing with your man on food issues. If you don't behave in an assertive way, like men everywhere who only take a firm attitude seriously, he just won't pay any attention to you.

Assertiveness on your part means stating the facts firmly without the anger that goes with an aggressive stance. You should make no small use of a sense of humor, cajoling, maybe stroking his ego a little bit—but never back off from your basic mission, which is to *convey essential information* about men's health to someone who is misinformed: *him.*

Not only will your assertive behavior benefit him in the long run (he may not be used to it from you and will resist at first), but you'll find that success with educating him will lead to a much-improved sense of self-esteem on your part. Many women who are involved with overweight men are, to some extent, "pleasers" in that they tend to avoid any kind of conflict as if it's the plague—especially with their man. Helping your man lose weight is a chance to change that behavior in yourself, as well as helping him lose weight.

CHAPTER FIVE

Where to Start

Once you've decided to help your man lose weight, you have to head in two directions: one is *practical*, the other *educational*.

THE PRACTICAL

The practical is fairly straightforward, and some of the work involved I've mentioned earlier in the book. You must:

- fat-proof your house, removing all high-fat toppings, rich desserts, and more than 30 percent fat foods from the house, along with sugary treats. Replace them with healthier substitutes (most low-fat, low-sugar foods can't be told from the original these days). Tell him what you're doing.
- exercise as much fat and sugar control as you can over what groceries come into the house.
- keep abreast of what new low-fat foods, fat substitutes, and sugar substitutes are coming on the market—it seems like there's a new high-quality one every other week. Store managers and grocery clerks are particularly helpful in this regard.

- use the 30-day Meal Plan outlined in Chapter 7 as the basis for your home food selections. It's designed for the average American male's high-fat taste buds but, if followed closely, it will bring his weight down without requiring him to change his eating habits overmuch.
- introduce the quietly effective exercise principles—they're designed to benefit you as much as him, because American couples on the whole get far too little in the way of physical exercise—in Chapter 8.

THE EDUCATIONAL

The educational aspect of helping your man lose weight takes a bit more finesse on your part, and that's where your perhaps underused assertive nature comes into play.

SUE JEFFRIES

After I realized that Ron's health was at risk because of all the weight he'd picked up between the time we got married and our fifteenth anniversary, I decided to get into the act, because he wasn't doing anything about it, and the delicate hints I tried— like mentioning the fact that I'd had the tailor let his pants out twice in the last six months—weren't working.

So I just started talking about food, about what was good, what was bad. I presented it all as though it were a discovery I'd made and I was just happy to know and benefit from it and I wanted him to as well. But while I didn't lecture him or whine, I didn't soft pedal anything I'd found out, about heart attacks and what caused them in men or anything else. I was a little bit apprehensive about how he'd react, whether he'd be bored or irritated, and although he was a little bit quiet at first, he didn't leave the table. . . . He listened, so I guess his weight might have been on his mind, too. I never did find out. We had a pretty good relationship, common interests and all that, and he started to get interested himself, asking questions. After a few months, he'd lost about 20 pounds and he was telling *me* things about women and nutrition. The only thing he really had *no* interest in, though, was cooking the food himself, if it involved more than opening the microwave door and setting the timer.

Sue's comments say it all, or at least most of it. She was assertive without being aggressive, she imparted knowledge to her man without anger and she didn't drop the subject when he didn't take to what she was saying immediately. And, as is usually the case with a couple that have a basically good relationship, the dialogue that Sue started with Ron about nutrition eventually become a two-way conversation, and in the end the need for him to lose weight become a means of further cementing their relationship.

WHEN TO TALK

With all your newfound knowledge about men and nutrition, you might wonder what the best time is to bring up the subject to him.

Men are best approached with nutritional information at mealtime or when you talk about going out to dinner. That's a good time to start discussing men's special medical problems and what can be done about them. Keep the conversation general at first, and gradually bring his personal experience into it. The important thing is to keep all references to his weight and to whatever problems result from it free of anger or derision. You should make it clear to him from your tone that you've learned these things out of concern for him. And don't overdo it! Know when to let the subject go for the moment (ten-minute lectures will turn him off; a two-minute infomercial of your own is far more effective).

THAT OLD DEVIL: LUNCH

Although your man will not respond to an angry, nagging tone, he will respond to a good-natured contest, and you can turn that to your advantage when dealing with the great stumbling block in any man's diet, his workday lunch. Men who are CEOs of corporations and men digging ditches all tend to commit major dietary sins at the midday meal. And they are experts at self-deception about what they're eating. Lunches, along with snacking, are a very significant source of excess male pounds.

When women tell me that they're perplexed about what they can do because their man isn't losing weight, despite the fact that they've fat-proofed the house and are following the eating plan, I suggest that they make a bet with him about what he eats for lunch and what it's doing to his waistline. The crux of the wager is that he has to make a list of what he eats when he's not at home during the day—and he has to be honest. If it's over 30 percent from fat, he has to pay you $50. Nine times out of ten, that list will come back looking like this, depending on whether or not he's on an expense account:

Lunch, Tuesday

prime rib
mashed potato with gravy
4 slices of bread with butter
coffee with apple pie
or
¼ pound cheeseburger
French fries
Soft drink

Looking at both food lists and doing a quick tally of approximately how much fat is in them (50 percent to 60 percent calories from fat)—along with what you've already told him that fat is doing to him—should be enough to persuade him that he has to change his midday eating habits. But the payoff is that it isn't really much of a change: all he has to do is switch his menu to:

flank steak with Worcestershire sauce
baked potato with low-fat sour cream
salad with lite vinegar and oil dressing

That's not a perfect meal, but portions being the same, the latter lunch has about half the fat his traditional one does—and it's the meat 'n potatoes taste he likes and is used to.

BARRY STREIBER

I finally ended up keeping a little notebook listing everything I ate during the course of a day, just to prove that my wife was wrong about where I was picking up pounds. I guess I thought they were coming out of thin air. Anyway, when I read the list at the end of the first week, I wondered where I found time to do any work, there was so much eating going on—and I was the one doing it. There's nothing like seeing it in black and white to convince you that you're wrong.

MAN AND GROCERY SHOPPING

Some food buying experience and lessons in label reading are also useful in educating a man and helping him lose weight—first with your help and then on his own. How to get him to do it? Well, in this case I'll go against my own general advice and say that a little bit of subterfuge may be a good thing when you're trying to get him to go food shopping with you. Tell him you need his help carrying the bags if the old "you should know what you're eating" argument doesn't work. Even one visit will help make him more food literate: you can point out the fat listings on labels (these will be standardized by order of Congress beginning in mid-1992) and my bet is that he will become absorbed—in much the same way that a car owner's manual can interest him—in the various tricks that food manufacturers play (my favorite is the "No Cholesterol" claim on products like potato chips that are sky-high in fat).

You don't have to be a nutrition expert in order to acquaint him with what's good and what's bad: just let him know the basic facts that you've learned in your years of buying food.

YOU AS JULIA CHILD

Yes, believe it or not, a man can learn something about cooking, in the "hands on" sense of preparing some dishes himself, and you can be the teacher. Don't make the mistake of thinking he's incapable of mastering the basics, and don't think you're going to turn him into the next master of the Cordon Bleu, either. All he has to know are some of the things that affect him directly, such as the difference between frying and broiling, how you can use Pam or some other substitute instead of butter when you're cooking, and how all the new low-fat prepared foods and fat substitutes (like Simplesse) can fit neatly with the kinds of things he likes to eat.

OUT ON THE TOWN

The other area you might have some problems with during the first few months after you start your man on a weight-reduction program are your nights out together. What, after all, can you do about fat when he suggests going out on the town, be it to a five-star restaurant or the great pizza joint on the corner?

The best scenario would be that all your hard work telling him about the benefits of low-fat, low-sugar, low-alcohol nutrition would kick into gear and he'll order just the right thing. But there's always a risk that won't happen. I suggest you not take the chance by jumping at the invitation (or suggesting an outing yourself) and that you then fix a low-fat, high-carbohydrate snack (say, plain bread with low-fat cheese like mozzarella, or a simple pasta salad) for the two of you before you leave the house. That way, he'll order less food when he gets to the restaurant because high-carbohydrate foods will fill him up quickly without blowing him up with fat.

YOU CAN LEAD A HORSE TO WATER . . .

As I've pointed out, if your man shows at least some interest in what you have to say, after a few months or so you won't have to give more than the occasional gentle reminder to him when he's fixing himself a snack or ordering in a restaurant. Unless there are deep-seated emotional problems underlying his overeating, he will actually begin to lose the taste for fat, and his body will respond to his improved eating by not producing the massive amount of bile salts needed to digest a high-fat, high-sugar diet.

SAM WATSON

Fat was my life, once upon a time. I used to down three eggs at breakfast with five strips of bacon, then I'd have a couple of cheeseburgers and fries at lunch and some kind of fatty red meat or pork at dinner. When my wife and I made a decision that it was time for me to lose, I was 50 or so pounds overweight, so I didn't have to go on one of those drastic diets for the really huge guys.

It wasn't easy at first, but after I'd slimmed down a little bit, I found that not only psychologically but *physically* my body didn't want to go back to my old habits. The one time I slid off my diet at a baseball game and ate three hot dogs—that would have been just an appetizer two years before—I just felt *very* uncomfortable for the next few hours. How do I say this without being gross? It was very similar to what happens when you mistakenly put bacon grease down your kitchen drain: plugged up.

HEALTH IN PRINT

I'd suggest that you also enlist an at-home ally in your campaign to educate him: the mailbox. Consider subscribing to the many general health magazines or newsletters that have sprung up around the country. But whatever you do, don't put anything with pictures of men who look like they spend half their lives in gymnasiums in front of him. That won't do anything but make him feel defeated before he gets into the fray. Don't think these publications are for doctors only—along with the fitness craze of the 1980s have come many magazines that are designed for the average reader.

But in the end, although you can inform him, help him, support him in every way and provide the spark that will put him on the road to better health, you can't trick, threaten, or force him to do it. His basic problem is that he's not been educated about how food and eating habits affect his health, and with this book you can help him bridge that gap. If you try all the things we've talked about and you still encounter hostility and stubbornness, in my opinion he likely has more complicated problems that require a professional's help. Unfortunately, serious medical complications due to his weight may have to emerge before he'll seek treatment.

But if you have a good relationship that's being threatened only by his lack of knowledge, you'll find that the role I've outlined for you in his weight loss will do much to cement your relationship. But before we plunge into the meat and potatoes of my 30-Day Meal plan, let's examine the special—and dangerous—role of sugar and of alcohol in a man's diet; a role with which almost all men (and most women) are unfamiliar.

CHAPTER SIX

Sugar and Alcohol Blues

Few women—and even fewer men—have any idea of the special role sugar and alcohol play in a man's weight gain. Neither do most doctors, whether they're weight-reduction specialists like myself or cardiologists. Oh, they may advise against eating certain sugary foods and drinking too much as obvious sources of extra calories (as well as other health problems ranging from tooth decay to alcoholism), but most fail to identify the two together as the root cause of a daily eating pattern that results not only in weight gain, but also in a psychological state that makes living with a man difficult.

OUR NATIONAL SWEET TOOTH

Americans in general eat too much refined sugar—if you divide up our sugar consumption by individual, every man, woman and child in the country downs a median of 105 pounds annually. That's a *median* figure, taking into account all those who don't eat any sugar at all. You can imagine what the figures are for obese men and women.

Frankly, although it's changing for the better, our food-manufacturing industry makes all this sugar intake a lot more likely: If you take a quick look at almost any label, you'll find sugar in one form or another listed as a significant ingredient. Ketchup and many prepared and frozen foods contain liberal dollops of sugar, although it's often disguised as fructose, sucrose, honey-sweetened, fruit-juice sweetened, mannitol, or sorbitol. The words may sound sweeter to the ear, but they're all the same simple carbohydrate, they all break down in the body to form the same substance—*blood glucose*, or blood sugar—which we rely on for energy.

The formation of glucose (sugar isn't our only source of it, other foods are converted to glucose as part of our normal digestive process) in our bodies is a perfectly natural and normal process, and simple sugars do have a place in a modern diet—in moderation. It's when *excessive* sugar intake becomes a part of your man's daily eating pattern that his weight gain is exacerbated by a chronic sugar-related condition called "reactive hypoglycemia." And though this form of hypoglycemia does affect women, too, in my experience it develops far more frequently in men because of their traditional eating habits.

REACTIVE HYPOGLYCEMIA AND DIABETES

These two afflictions are often confused and thought similar because of the sugar connection, but actually their opposites. Diabetes, a complicated, life-threatening disease, is due to the presence of *too much* sugar in the blood. Diabetics do not produce enough insulin in their pancreas to get their glucose from blood to cell, thus starving their body of energy. With hypoglycemia, too *little* sugar in the blood causes problems. For overweight men, the two form a double whammy: The overweight man will often progress from hypoglycemia to diabetes if he's overweight for many years. His body's reaction is fairly simple: after years of producing too much insulin, it gets worn out; as a result, it doesn't produce enough insulin to open the cell doors (receptor sites) to allow the glucose to enter and go to work as energy. Heredity, of course, plays a role, though the medical community can't say exactly what. Suffice it to say that if your man's father was overweight, and ate a great deal of sugar—like father, like son. But if his father was skinny as a rail and a vegetarian, that doesn't mean your man won't have a problem.

MEN'S UPS AND DOWNS WITH SUGAR

Whatever kind of sugar a man ends up eating, from "natural sweeteners" to plain old cane sugar, it all ends up in the same place—his bloodstream. His body converts all types of sugar into glucose, or blood sugar, that his cells use as fuel. The fuel actually enters the cell courtesy of insulin, a substance produced by the pancreas that's a kind of go-between for the body; it acts as the key to cells, permitting blood glucose to be used as energy instead of being converted to and stored as fat. A man's normal fasting blood sugar level, on a diet with moderate sugar intake (this figure is correct for both men and women) is about 90 to 100 milligrams per deciliter of blood.

When a man eats a single highly sweetened snack, like a sugar-glazed donut, his blood glucose level may suddenly shoot up to 170 to 180 milligrams in a matter of minutes. This is another problem with sweet foods: the sugar in them is digested much more quickly than are other nutrients, and the result is that the body falls under the mistaken impression that it has to get fuel to cells quickly. This elevated glucose level causes his pancreas to work overtime producing enough insulin to cope with the unexpected supply of blood sugar. A 170 to 180 level is not something I like to see, but his body can cope with it. It's when he starts eating large amounts of sugar on a daily basis that he'll begin to have more serious problems.

For example, if he eats the equivalent of two Snickers bars or a standard-sized banana split, his blood sugar will really shoot sky-high in short order—up to and maybe a little bit past the 200 milligram mark. A signal will go from brain to pancreas to produce more insulin to get all this sugar out of the bloodstream and into the cells. The cells are reluctant to open their doors—they've already got a normal store of sugar and they don't need or want any more.

The pancreas responds by producing *three to four* times the normal amount of insulin it normally would. With this amount of insulin banging at the door, the cells finally open up and take the unwanted, unnecessary sugar. All this happens in pretty short order, and the quick lowering of blood sugar levels causes that hyper, nervous feeling he gets two to three hours after he's eaten too many sweets, because his blood glucose level, now below normal, is telling his brain that he is hungry. Eventually, though, he doesn't feel energetic, just kind of cranky—and hungry once again!

But after every peak there has to be a valley, and so too with sugar. His glucose level (remember, *blood glucose* and *blood sugar* are interchangeable terms) will begin to drop in the first half hour after the insulin has done its work, but it *won't* return to a normal level; it will drop way down in the second thirty minutes after he's put his pancreas through the paces, to about 75 to 80 milligrams. What happens next? Not surprisingly, his brain's hypothalamus, which controls appetite, gets a message from the rest of the body saying "feed me," because there's not a normal level of sugar in the blood, too much of it has gone to the cells. The typical 30- to 40-pound overweight adult man will respond by eating even *more* sugar, usually in combination with some kind of fat, which will satisfy him for the moment.

Then comes the real hitch: after this feeding, his pancreas has to produce *five to six* times the normal amount of insulin to get his cells to take the glucose in his blood. They succeed, but then comes an even worse crash. His blood sugar level will drop to 50 or even 40 milligrams, making him irritable, jumpy, and ravenously hungry for more of the same bad food.

And, in the typical American household, that's just about the time that he walks in the front door, looking for dinner.

HIS DAILY PATTERN

As a boy, I remember being fascinated by the fact that my dad could dash out of the house every morning with just a cup of coffee and still be a "big"—meaning overweight—guy. Years later, as a doctor, I realized that his morning ritual marked the beginning of a daily pattern that does much to keep so many men past thirty on a nasty dangerous cycle of overeating. See if this sounds familiar to you.

BREAKFAST—SORT OF

An at-home breakfast is often light or nonexistent for most overweight men. There's the quick cup of coffee, sometimes accompanied by a piece of toast (with butter and jam of course). Rarely will they eat a big breakfast.

THE MORNING SNACK ATTACK

But then on his way to work, he'll stop to get a bag of donuts (and I mean a *bag*, the kind with grease showing through the sides, not some nutritious little muffin) or a heavy, fatty/sugary breakfast, like fast-food pancakes with syrup. He'll either wolf them down in the car or gobble them up quickly at the office. And if he doesn't (or isn't able) to buy a sugar/fat fix on his way to work, he'll make sure he gets one shortly after he arrives—either at the vending machine or down at the corner deli.

> TIM SAVEROW
>
> I used to *act* like I was in a hurry in the morning—deliberately coming downstairs late—so I could just gulp down a quick cup of coffee and dash out the door. Then I'd go straight to this great donut shop—The 'Nut Stop—a couple of blocks from work and buy a half-dozen of those sugar-coated raspberry jam–filled donuts and wash them down with a big cup of coffee. It sounds disgusting, but even now, after I've lost all this weight, I remember having a real feeling of satisfaction as I crumpled up the bag and tossed it in the wastebasket.

Tim's pattern is fairly typical. And with this dose of sugar, fat, and caffeine in the morning, the whole hypoglycemia chain reaction commences.

Soon after Tim finishes his morning fix, his sugar levels will go sky-high, but then with some overtime work by his pancreas, they come tumbling back down, making him hungry—just in time for lunch.

A LETHAL LUNCH

Whether he's eating a box lunch on a construction site, dining in an expensive steakhouse, or ordering out from the corner deli, a man with a weight problem comes to the midday meal with his appetite artificially fueled by his plummeting blood sugar levels. He will respond by overeating, and since he believes, as we discussed earlier, then there's nothing wrong with eating large amounts of food at one meal, he'll indulge himself in a big, fatty, sugary meal (remember all the hidden sugar in our food; many fast-food outlets even dip their French fries in a sugar syrup before freezing to "improve" their taste!) Examples:

Restaurant
more than 4 ounces of high-fat beef or pork
potato (any type) with butter and sour cream
slice of cheesecake
cocktail

Fast Food
hamburger or breaded, fat-fried chicken breast or fish
    fillet
French fries
salad bar—loaded with high-fat, creamy dressings
soft drink

Box Lunch
prepared meat sandwich (ham, veal loaf, etc.),
    slathered with mayonnaise and topped with
    high-fat cheese
bag of chips
package of cookies or cake dessert
soft drink

Now, these meals certainly have different price tags, but in terms of his health, they have the same effect—all are over 50 percent calories from fat.

A LATE AFTERNOON SUGAR RUN

After a couple of hours, his blood sugar will sink again, even lower than before, to 45 or 50 milligrams. Whether his job is high pressure, low pressure, or no pressure, he'll feel hyper, irritable, and perhaps a little bit faint, because his body is telling him to get his sugar levels up again. At about 3:30 or 4:00 he'll take a walk to the vending machine or walk down to the corner store and buy something with a heavy dose of . . . sugar. Wham! He's happy again—for a short while.

WHERE'S DINNER???

Because that late afternoon dose of sugar didn't have nearly enough fat in it to satisfy the hunger that repeated injections of sugar are causing, he's ravenous and often in a close-to-unreasonable state by the time he gets home. That's why so often a man demands his dinner the moment he gets in the door—and if he doesn't get it, he'll hang around the kitchen, maybe eating right out of the pot, until he does.

This is the time of day when alcohol comes into play as well. If he can't get dinner right away, the overweight man will often get himself a beer or cocktail. Alcohol is the perfect quick-fix solution to his problem: unlike other sugars, which need to go to the small intestine to be absorbed, it is absorbed directly from the stomach, since, being a simple carbohydrate, it acts very much like a *simple* sugar. And so it satisfies that craving, and it also anesthetizes—all too temporarily—the appetite center in the brain. So it calms him down. But again, in an hour or so he'll be ready to wolf down even more food.

JANE FARBER

My post-work life with Phil just got to be a bad joke. I left my job at 4:00 P.M., and he'd get home at 5:30, so I got something together for dinner. Now, everyday wasn't a holiday for me— I'm working in the public school system—but with Phil, he'd come home looking like he was really in *pain* until he had dinner. It got so I didn't bother cooking anything creative anymore: he was just concerned about *volume,* and his own was expanding, mainly around the waistline. Then he'd doze off in front of the television, wake up at 9:00 or 10:00, have a bowl of ice cream and conk out again. I mean, it wasn't like I expected to go out ballroom dancing every night, but I would have liked a little conversation. All I'd get is my head taken off if dinner wasn't ready.

SWEET DREAMS?

No, the cycle doesn't end with dinner. I'll bet my bottom dollar that, like Jane Farber's husband, your man will fix himself one more snack, either full of fat or both fat and sugar (I've heard of men who eat bologna sandwiches piled with mustard and mayo—or thick peanut butter and jelly sandwiches—at 10:00 or 11:00) before he gives out for the night. Then, with a belly full of fat and sugar (a full stomach keeps blood circulating around *it,* rather than the brain; that's why he dozes after eating), he'll sleep through until morning—then start the whole cycle over again.

With severe cases of reactive hypoglycemia, however even his sleep patterns can be severely disrupted. A day of volatile sugar ups and downs can cause his blood sugar to drop like a stone while he sleeps, causing him to go into a kind of "sugar coma" which some researchers believe contributes to the possibility of heart attack or stroke. Although these severe cases of hypoglycemia are relatively rare and occur mainly in men over fifty, even a younger man is laying the groundwork for poor health if he is abusing sugar.

THE MAN-SUGAR-WEIGHT CONNECTION

You're probably wondering how his daily sugar routine directly affects your man's weight. This is the point where everything we've talked about concerning men, their lifelong habits and their post-thirty physiology come into play.

The male pattern I've just traced, one that you've probably observed without fully understanding, is a surefire way for him to gain weight. He's eating sugar in massive amounts, causing the so-called brain appestat controlling his hunger to be stimulated artificially. He will sometimes eat *more* sugar to satisfy that urge, or drink coffee, and the two substances will combine to make him extra irritable—and even hungrier. When it comes time for him to eat his midday or evening meal, his early socialization will kick in and he'll wolf down far larger amounts of (usually fatty) food than his sedentary body will ever use. Taking full advantage of his slowing metabolism, the fat from these forced feedings will just collect around his chest and middle. That's another side effect of reactive hypoglycemia in a man: he's so exhausted from riding on this twenty-four-hour sugar roller coaster that he has no energy for exercise or any other physical activity.

MAN AND SEROTONIN

A natural brain chemical, serotonin, also plays a role in his sugar consumption, mood and weight gain.

Serotonin plays a key role in giving us our sense of well-being; it's an organic pleasure substance and the brain maintains a constant, moderate flow of it. Use of cocaine, in fact, overstimulates the brain's production of serotonin, resulting in the exaggerated sense of being "on top of the world" that drug abusers seek. Serotonin is a kind of natural drug, production of which can be encouraged or inhibited by dietary factors, like sugar intake.

When blood sugar levels drop below 100 milligrams, as his does when he crashes after lunch and just before dinner, serotonin production in his brain is inhibited as a result of a long chain of complicated physiological reactions. That's when he gets grumpy, until he has the sugar fix that will start the serotonin pumping again.

By five o'clock, then, you're facing the results of his overeating

sugar, artificially induced hunger pangs, restricted serotonin production—and probably a couple of cups of coffee thrown in to run
his nervous system extra raw.

WHY HYPOGLYCEMIA DOESN'T AFFECT YOU

Again, we come back to learned eating habits to explain why
women are so rarely affected by this form of hypoglycemia. It's really
pretty simple.

Women, even if they have a weight problem, tend to eat small
amounts of food (even if it's fatty) at intervals throughout the day.
Whatever other problems with weight your eating habits may cause
you, you definitely *do not* suffer from the bouncing blood sugar that
contributes so much to *his* waistline, because you don't ingest large
amounts of sugary, fatty foods on a regular—daily—basis.

GRETA CALDWELL

Living with my brother, who was about 80 pounds overweight, was a great education in men's eating habits for me,
because I've never lived with a man, except when I was growing
up. Luther always wanted to eat these *big meals*, which I had no
interest in whatsoever. Even if we were having a microwave
meal, he'd always heat up at least two meals for himself, while
I'd have half of one. It's not as though I was starving myself; he
just seemed frenetic about really *stuffing* himself. There was
something *unnatural* about how hungry he was at night. And
he'd just read and go to sleep by 10:00, so he wasn't working it
off in any way.

It's not that you don't ever experience sugar ups and downs: I
haven't yet met a woman who hasn't downed a pint of Häagen-Dazs
at least once, felt the immediate joy of the experience and the sugar
crash shortly afterward. The wonderful thing about a woman's eating habits is that she doesn't eat sugar every day, she doesn't eat it
in combination with large amounts of fatty foods, and she is not on
a cycle that leads her to do it again.

IS SUGAR ADDICTIVE FOR MEN?

Yes, the overweight man often has a sugar habit that meets the clinical description of addiction. Sugar alters his mood (causing wild swings), can adversely affect his job performance and his relationship with people. His life is being ruled by a substance. I've even seen severely overweight men whose need for sugar is so great that, despite the health risk, they'll eat it anyway, against doctor's orders, stashing it around the house, much as an alcoholic might hide liquor bottles, or a substance abuser, drugs.

JOYCE ARENS

When Harry's weight finally caused him to have a heart attack, he ended up in the hospital for three weeks. While he was there I used his car to go to work. That's when I started finding the candy wrappers: under the spare tire in the car, in the glove compartment—anywhere but on the seat or in the house where I could see them. He even had a bag of those mini-Baby Ruths, the kind you give to kids on Halloween, stuck in the back of the tool cabinet out in the garage. I could tell they were fairly fresh, and that he'd kept on eating them despite what the doctor said.

THE SUGAR AND ALCOHOL CONNECTION

I've already told you that alcohol is metabolized (or used by the body) as a simple sugar, and it contributes to the whole reactive hypoglycemia cycle, albeit in a different way than candy and other sugar-filled foods. And in combination with standard-issue sweets, alcohol can cause twice the problems.

There are men who will substitute alcoholic drinks for some sweet foods, not so much from love of alcohol as for the combination of sugar in the drink and the calming effect the drink has after a sugar-exacerbated stress-filled day (and so it becomes a quick fix for stress and for sugar cravings).

Liquor, even seemingly moderate amounts, will wreak havoc

on your man's attempt to lose weight. A single 12-ounce beer contains 150 calories (light has 100) while hard liquor has as many calories as it does proof (100 proof—100 calories per ounce). Among men whose business takes them into restaurants or around bars and nightclubs a lot, it's not uncommon to have more than two or three drinks a day. That means that 30 to 40 percent of their calories are coming from the simple sugars of alcohol, and alcohol has no nutrients: they're so-called empty calories.

Alcohol works to expand a man's waistline in more than one way, though. The sugar in it has the same effect on his appetite that a candy bar does, with the added effect of anesthetizing his appetite control center—for a brief time. Within an hour after he has one or two beers or as many cocktails, his hunger pangs will be twice as bothersome as they were before. To make things worse, a drink or two just before dinner is served will help dampen what few inhibitions about overeating he might have, or he may forget how much he's eaten. Result? Even more food goes down his hatch.

HOW MUCH HE'LL GAIN

A man with 30 to 40 pounds of extra weight will tend toward diets that consist of 2,000 calories of simple sugar and 1,500 or so calories of fat and protein. Since his basal metabolic rate—the average rate at which he burns fat calories as energy (if he's not exercising regularly)—is probably about 2,900 calories, that leaves 600 calories waiting around for something to do. And whether those calories are from sugar, protein or fat, they'll get their marching orders from his brain very shortly: *convert to fat and head for storage,* most likely around his waist or chest. Repeated on a daily basis, this whole sorry chain of events can easily put 3 to 4 pounds a month on him.

HELPING HIM BREAK THE SUGAR HABIT

Two of the most difficult aspects of getting a man to give up his sugar and afterwork (or lunch) cocktail habits (the latter sacrifice can be temporary) are: 1) your man doubtless has no idea how sugar is affecting him day to day; and 2) when he does realize what's going on with his body, he'll be afraid, as many addictive personalities are, that he *won't be able* to do without his daily dose of sugar and alcohol.

ADDRESS THE ISSUE

As I said in the last chapter, when you're trying to convey medical facts, it's best to take an assertive stance and talk about the problem with him directly. One way to prove you're right, without gloating, is to trace his dietary day for him, something on the order of, "And then at about 3:00 or 4:00 in the afternoon, I'll bet you have some kind of snack. . . ." This approach prevents denial on his part—no convenient memories—and will convince him you know what you're talking about. So now he's informed.

FEARS OF THE SUGARLESS

Whatever you do, don't leave a void when it comes to buying sweet foods—if you completely shut him off from them, he'll just go out and buy them himself, despite the fact that he knows how harmful they are. All he cares about is that he doesn't like how he feels when he doesn't have them.

You'd be wise to buy nonfat, high-fiber, naturally sweetened cookies as well as sugarless mints and gums, and make sure he has some with him at all times. A little real sugar in a high-fiber cookie is absorbed slowly and gets the serotonin levels back up, especially at the critical time of 4:00 P.M. (It's similar to substituting methadone for heroin.) And using non-fat, low-calorie snacks that have complex carbohydrates will contribute to his breaking the hypoglycemia habit. You'll notice that I *don't* recommend hard sugarless candies: I don't believe in them. They are usually sweetened with mannitol or sorbitol, two man-made substances which, though, they're not sugars, strictly speaking, end up fueling his hypoglycemic fire in much the same way real sugars do.

THE FOUR O'CLOCK KEY

Dealing successfully with the powerful sugar craving your man feels late in the afternoon is the most important key to controlling his reactive hypoglycemia. Most of the time, unfortunately, you're not there. But you can supply him with a solution that doesn't require him to suffer and which will let him lose weight.

TIM SMEGELSKI

My wife and I both went on a special diet a couple of years ago, when I first developed a heart problem. It went okay the first couple of weeks, but then I started feeling depressed a lot of the time. It wasn't so much the taste of the food I missed—I think all that sugar and fat I had been eating actually made me feel better.

Tim is right: it *did* make him feel good by pumping up his serotonin levels. But he would have succeeded on that first diet if he had just not cut out both sugar and fat cold turkey.

The ideal solution is to eat something in the late afternoon that's both sweet (flavored with either a small amount of fruit juice, honey, fructose, or even sucrose) and full of fiber, like an oatmeal-raisin cookie with fruit juice or something similar. The sweet taste and small amount of natural sugar will tell the brain that it's getting a destructive dose of sugar when it's really getting just enough to keep the serotonin levels up. And the fiber will stay in the stomach longer than sugar or fat, making your man less ravenous at dinnertime.

There are a number of these juice-sweetened cookies on the market now, but inspect the label carefully to make sure there is no added fat and the dietary fiber is relatively high. Cookies with oats or other grains near the top of the ingredients list are your best bet.

If you don't have the cookies available to you, dried fruit of any kind is a good, sweet, fiber-filled alternative to junk sweets. And although it is important to clean any dried fruit from one's teeth soon after eating (the fruit sugars stick to the enamel and form plaque and tartar very quickly), it's a lot cheaper to buy a new toothbrush and some dental floss than it is to undergo a triple bypass because excess weight has caused heart problems.

OFF THE SAUCE

Handling the boozy end of the *sugar + alcohol = pounds* equation is a little bit easier for you and your man, provided that an alcohol-abuse problem doesn't exist. After you make him aware of the far-reaching effect of alcohol on his weight, you should begin stocking a lot of diet drinks of all types in the house. Ask him, just as an experiment, not to drink during the workday or with friends immediately afterward. Near-beers and "alcohol-free" wines don't do the trick. In fact, they're not completely alcohol-free; there's a trace amount in them that can spark the desire for more, and the sugar in them can also set off the hypoglycemia dominoes. Best of all, once he gets off his weight-gaining, hypoglycemic eating pattern, he can have a beer, a drink, or a glass of wine once in a while, as you'll see in the eating plan given in the next chapter.

PART TWO

A PLAN
OF ACTION

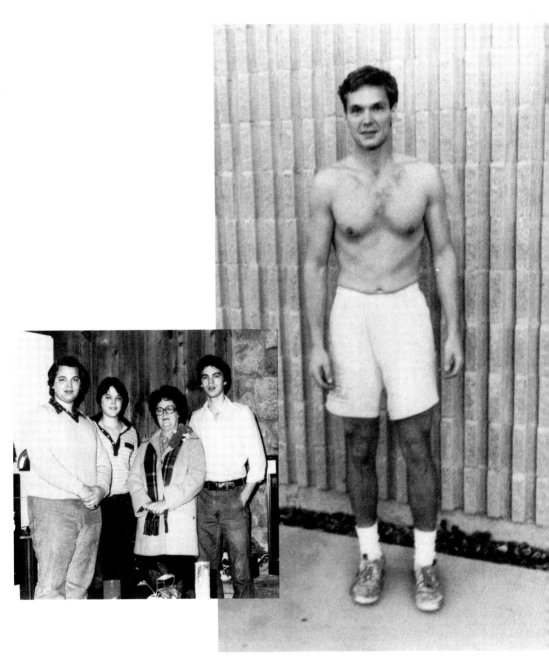

RONALD H., Denver, CO
Before: 298 pounds
After: 165 pounds
Total lost: 133 pounds

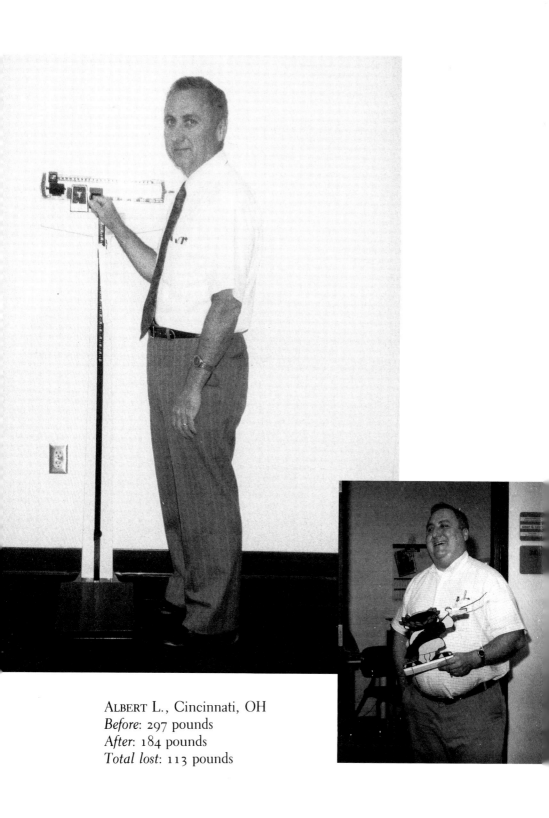

ALBERT L., Cincinnati, OH
Before: 297 pounds
After: 184 pounds
Total lost: 113 pounds

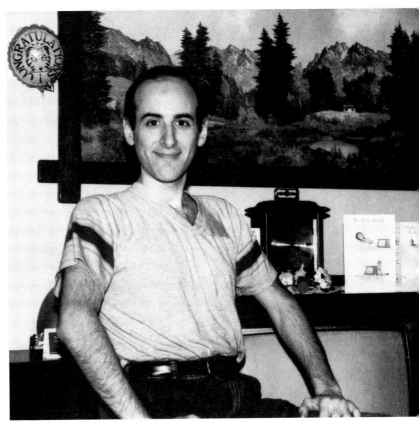

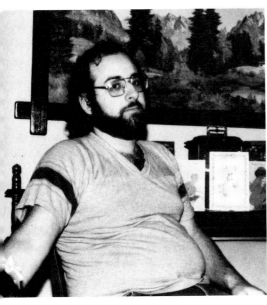

John P., Bellerose, NY
Before: 212 pounds
After: 145 pounds
Total lost: 67 pounds

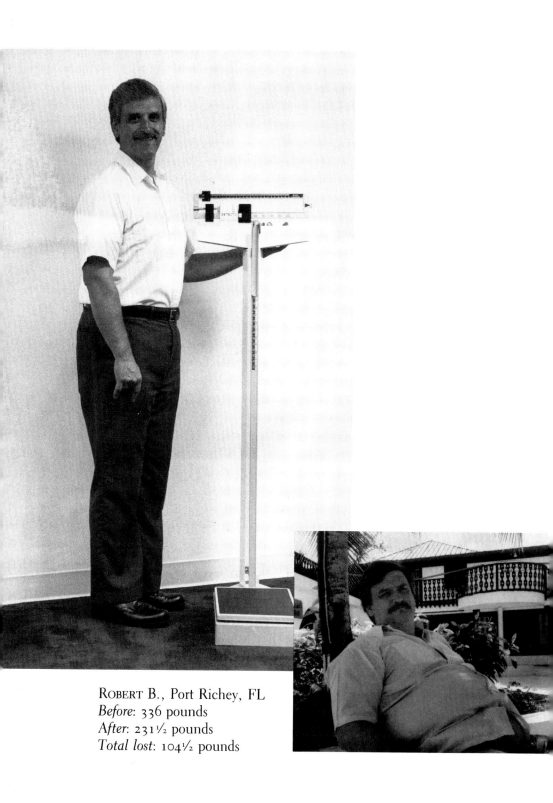

ROBERT B., Port Richey, FL
Before: 336 pounds
After: 231½ pounds
Total lost: 104½ pounds

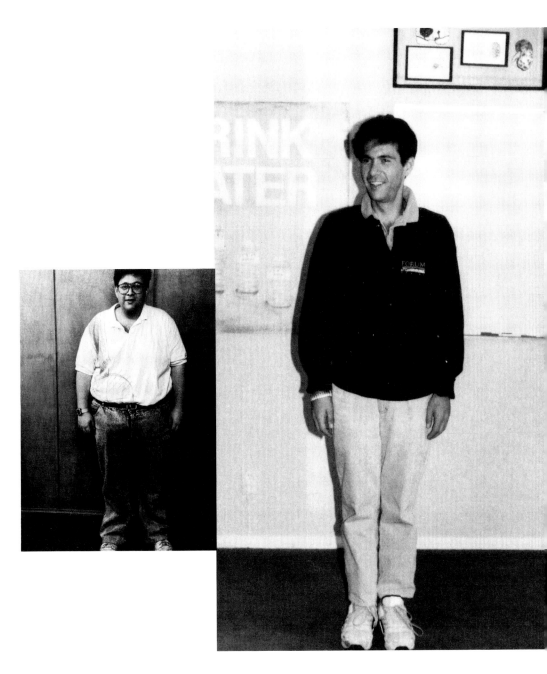

JEFF G., Sherman Oaks, CA
Before: 330 pounds
After: 155 pounds
Total lost: 175 pounds

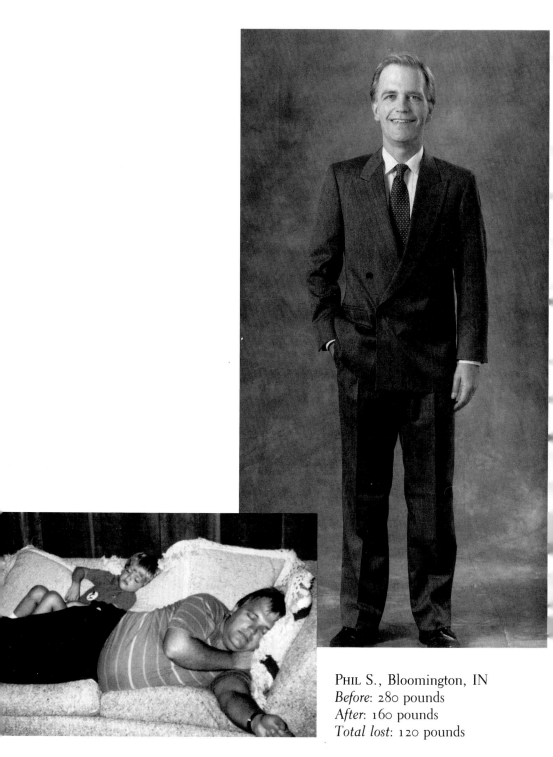

PHIL S., Bloomington, IN
Before: 280 pounds
After: 160 pounds
Total lost: 120 pounds

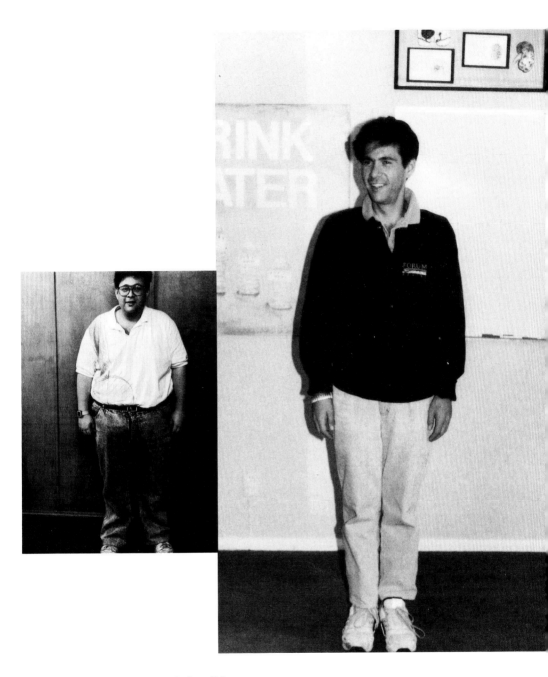

JEFF G., Sherman Oaks, CA
Before: 330 pounds
After: 155 pounds
Total lost: 175 pounds

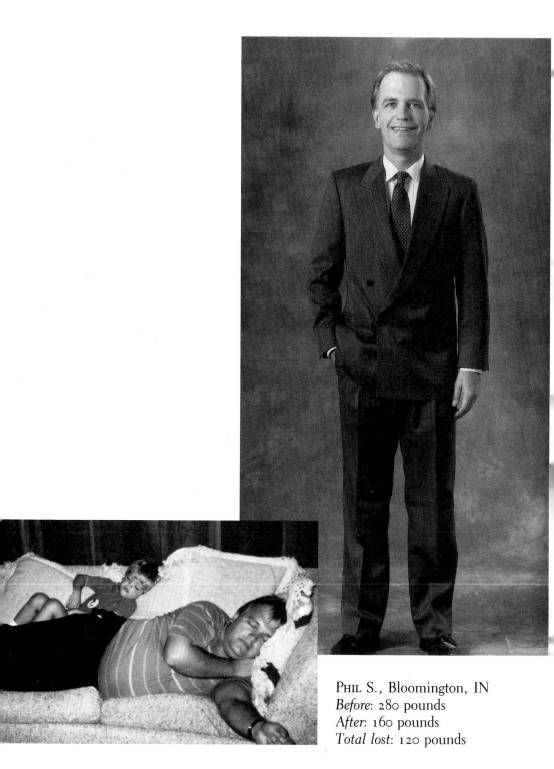

Phil S., Bloomington, IN
Before: 280 pounds
After: 160 pounds
Total lost: 120 pounds

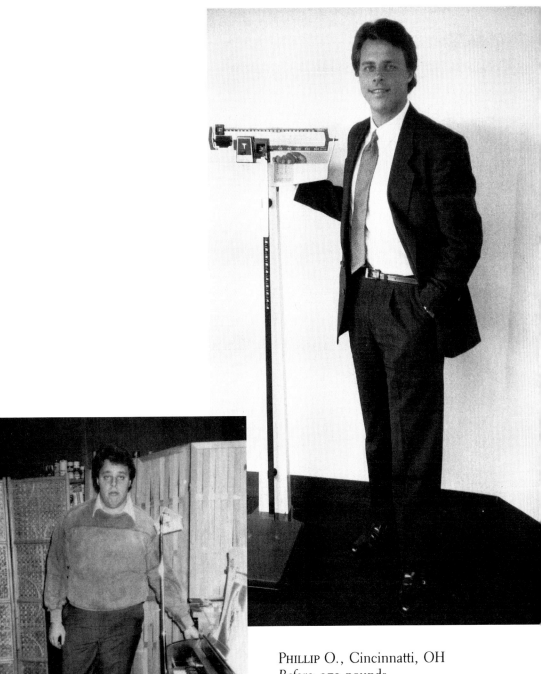

PHILLIP O., Cincinnatti, OH
Before: 273 pounds
After: 168 pounds
Total lost: 105 pounds

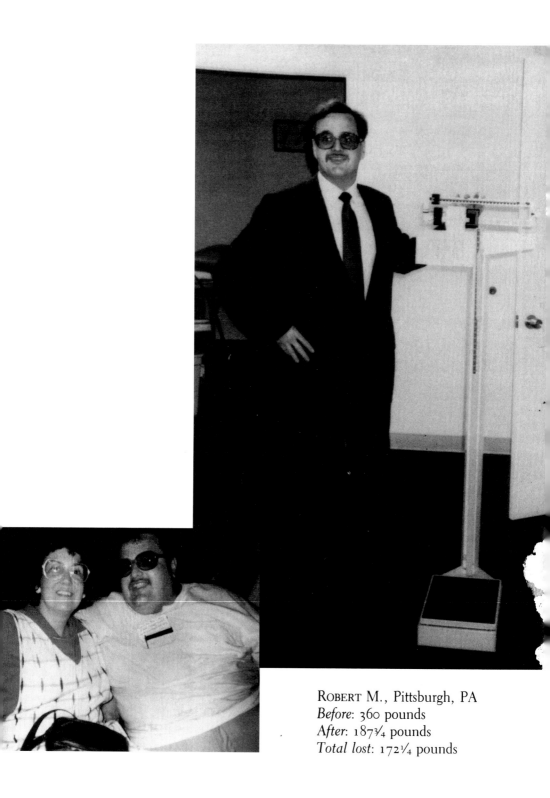

ROBERT M., Pittsburgh, PA
Before: 360 pounds
After: 187¾ pounds
Total lost: 172¼ pounds

CHAPTER SEVEN

The 30-Day Weight-Loss Program

Most people would find the "perfect diet" pretty boring. But men, especially, fear dietary change and are loath to eat anything that has even a hint of the healthy about it. So even after you've educated your man as to the dangers of male overweight, you'll face a dilemma in deciding how to prepare meals that will help him lose which also appeal to him. Because you can bet that unless he's really under a death threat from a doctor, if you try to put him on cottage cheese, pita bread, skinless chicken, and mineral water, he'll be back to fatty steaks, potatoes, and gravy in a flash.

WHAT HE'LL EAT

In helping your man lose weight, you should try to strike a balance among carbohydrates, proteins, and fats. Years ago, the emphasis of professional nutritionists was on proteins, but now there's been a shift to carbohydrates as a more ideal food.

That doesn't change the fact that your man's palate is probably accustomed to a traditional American diet, which is high in fat and 95 sugar, and low in grains and carbohydrates. And while there's often plenty of protein in the typical man's diet, it usually comes wrapped in fat. As you now know, changing these deeply ingrained habits—in women as well as men—is the most difficult part of instituting and then maintaining a healthy body. So the question is: How do you let him eat what he likes, and what he's accustomed to, and still help him to lose?

MODERN TECHNOLOGY

Fortunately, the American food industry, while lacking in many other areas, has responded fairly well to the public's desire for low-fat foods—in fact, more than 1,000 new low-fat products went on the market in 1990 alone.

In another improvement, as of mid-1992, the Food and Drug Administration (FDA) will clamp down on misleading food label claims. Gone will be those "No Cholesterol" banners on products that are full of fat and never had any cholesterol to begin with. Banished as well will be the "85% Fat-free" claims, when the product really contains 60 to 70 percent calories from fat, more than *twice* what the government's minimal standards for good nutrition suggest as everyone's maximum: 30 percent. The FDA will also require companies manufacturing products that don't currently list all their ingredients to provide greater detail, so you, as a consumer, can know what's in them before you buy. And although the new rules are far from perfect, almost all food products will have an important new addition: they will list the percentage in one serving of calories that come from fat.

THE 30-DAY MEAL PLAN

All of these changes make formulating an eating plan designed for men a little bit easier. Many of their favorite foods (meats, cheeses, desserts) are now available in quality low-fat versions. Again, if we were to have my way, we'd all be eating some skinless chicken, drinking mineral water, having fresh vegetables, lots of carbohydrates—and less than 12 percent of our calories would come from fat. But very few men would stick to that particular meal plan, so a different approach is in order.

The 30-Day Meal Plan provides that different approach: Your man will still have many of the familiar everyday foods—not "diet food"—but if they're low-fat, he's capable of losing 1 to 2 pounds per week (assuming that he's keeping up his daily walking routine as outlined in Chapter 8). By providing him with an average of 1,700 to 1,900 calories per day, he will burn considerably more than that. And for each daily plan, the total of calories from fat is less than 30 percent, even though individual meals may go a little bit higher.

A FOCUS ON FAT

The 30-Day Meal Plan doesn't have to be rigidly followed: You can mix and match the meals as you please, and I hope you'll add your own ideas as time goes by. My only requirement would be that you keep the fat below 30 percent for each meal. What the plan does is show you and the man in your life that he can go on eating pretty much as he used to, but with low-fat foods. And the more you buy of these foods, the more of them the food manufacturers will produce. Included in the plan are both home-cooked and prepared foods, even wise choices in fast-food restaurants. Eventually, I would hope that both of you will cut the fat in your diet even further, but for now I'll settle for that 30 percent mark.

Obviously, if you're preparing the food, you'll be eating it as well. The average woman not trying to lose should have nothing to worry about in terms of weight gain, if she doesn't snack excessively during the day. A woman trying to lose weight should reduce other-than-vegetable dishes by one-third in portion size for herself.

As approved by hospital nutritionist Dan Curtis, R.D., of St. Joseph's Hospital in Fullerton, California, the daily menus meet all

Recommended Daily Allowances (RDAs) of nutrients as determined by the United States Department of Agriculture, and contain a healthful amount of fiber as well. By my first concern—and I can't emphasize this enough—is to get his fat intake down. When you're mixing and matching and moving the meals around to prevent boredom, just give some thought to his taste buds as well as his waistline.

SUGAR

The 30-Day Meal Plan largely banishes sugar from his diet, although there is the occasional lapse with dessert. These are infrequent and shouldn't do him any real harm. I recommend nonrefined sugar or no-sugar substitute sweet snacks, such as dried fruit or sugarless gum. Some cookies are also acceptable. I have formulated a fruit-juice sweetened, high-fiber snack myself, All-Natural Honey Raisin Oatmeal Cookies, which I have found effectively satisfies the yen for sugar and helps break the carbo craver's cycle. It makes a good afternoon and evening snack, and is available in most grocery stores.

The following is a list of some snacks with which he can lose weight:

- Sugarless gum
- Dried Fruit
- Fresh fruit (bananas included)
- Fruit-juice sweetened, high-fiber cookies (such as All-Natural Honey Raisin Oatmeal Cookies)
- Air-popped popcorn (plain, moderate salt okay)
- Raw vegetable sticks with nonfat dressing

ALCOHOL

I haven't allowed for any alcohol in the plan, because I would prefer that he not have any. But men, being creatures of habit, will often have it no matter what I say. If he has a cocktail, glass of wine, or a couple of beers each week, it won't slow his progress any more than that will slow down his loss—especially if he's sitting having a drink instead of getting some exercise.

NUTRITIONAL GOALS

The 30-Day Meal Plan is not a diet, as such. It is an eating plan designed to take the weight off him. If he wants to fine tune by exploring other types of diets, supplements—even vegetarianism— more power to him. My goal is to help you help *him* get over those first psychological and taste-bud hurdles. What happens after that is entirely up to him.

THE 30-DAY MEAL PLAN

A WORD ABOUT BRAND NAMES

Throughout the 30-Day Meal Plan that follows, brand names are used from time to time. I have found these brands to be quality products, but that in no way precludes you from making your own choices at the market. But here's a legend for some brand names of products that come up fairly frequently in the meal plans.

- nonfat mayo: Kraft
- nonfat cheese, presliced: Kraft
- 98% fat-free ham: Danola
- Butter substitute: Butter Buds or Molly McButter
- Egg substitute: Egg Beaters
- lowest-fat margarine: Heart Beat—the only margarine called for in recipes
- nonfat high-fiber cookie: All-Natural Honey Raisin Oatmeal

NOTE: *The recipes for all asterisked items (*) follow the Meal Plan.*

DAY 1

BREAKFAST

HAM AND CHEESE OMELETTE*
2 slices 100% whole-wheat bread, toasted
2 teaspoons Heart Beat margarine (optional)
2 teaspoons sugar-free jelly
½ cup chopped fresh pineapple
Regular/decaf coffee or tea with Nutrasweet and/or 1% low-fat milk
> *Total Calories:* 418
> *Grams of Fat:* 11
> *Percent Calories from Fat:* 24

LUNCH

FAST-FOOD LUNCH
McLean Deluxe (or any generic lean hamburger that doesn't exceed 12 grams of fat)
Side salad
Nonfat dressing
Small orange juice
> *Total Calories:* 470
> *Grams of Fat:* 10
> *Percent Calories from Fat:* 19

DINNER

BARBECUED SHISH KEBAB*
½ cup steamed or boiled rice (Minute rice is okay)
Green salad
2 tablespoons nonfat dressing
1 whole-wheat roll
1 teaspoon Heart Beat margarine (for roll)
1 fresh peach, quartered
½ cup nonfat dairy frozen dessert, such as Simple Pleasures
> *Total Calories:* 599
> *Grams of Fat:* 12
> *Percent Calories from Fat:* 18

DAY 2

BREAKFAST
SCRAMBLED EGGS*
1 whole-grain English muffin (2 slices), toasted
2 teaspoons Heart Beat margarine
2 teaspoons sugar-free jelly
¼ cantaloupe
Regular/decaf coffee or tea with Nutrasweet, 1% low-fat milk
> *Total Calories: 398*
> *Grams of Fat: 10*
> *Percent Calories from Fat: 23*

LUNCH
LEAN HAM AND CHEESE SANDWICH
2 1-ounce slices 98% fat-free presliced deli ham
2 slices nonfat presliced cheese
1 tablespoon nonfat mayonnaise
Lettuce, tomato, and pickles
Noncreamy mustard
2 slices 100% whole-wheat bread

⅓ cantaloupe
12 Oat Thin crackers
> *Total Calories: 457*
> *Grams of Fat: 8*
> *Percent Calories from Fat: 16*

DINNER
FISH PLATE
6 ounces shark, broiled or barbecued
1 potato, baked
1 cup steamed or boiled carrot cubes
Butter substitute, such as Molly McButter
1 slice 100% whole-wheat bread
1 teaspoon Heart Beat margarine
1 slice watermelon
Raw Vegetable Salad
> 1–2 cups cut-up cucumber, lettuce, tomato, beets, or any
> other raw vegetables you prefer
> 3 tablespoons nonfat Ranch dressing
> ½ cup nonfat frozen yogurt
> *Total Calories: 777*
> *Grams of Fat: 9.5*
> *Percent Calories from Fat: 11*

DAY 3

CEREAL AND BAGEL

1½ cups wheat-flake cereal
1 whole banana, sliced crosswise
1 cup 1% low-fat milk

1 whole-grain bagel, toasted
2 tablespoons "light" Philadelphia Cream Cheese
2 teaspoons sugar-free strawberry jelly
Regular/decaf coffee or tea with Nutrasweet, 1% low-fat milk

> *Total Calories:* 600
> *Grams of Fat:* 10
> *Percent Calories from Fat:* 15

LUNCH
TOASTED TUNA SANDWICH

Combine:
1 6⅛-ounce can water-packed tuna
1 tablespoon nonfat mayonnaise
About 1 tablespoon each chopped celery and diced onion

2 slices oat-bran bread, toasted
Lettuce and sliced tomato

1 fresh green apple
8 Ritz crackers

> *Total Calories:* 532
> *Grams of Fat:* 13
> *Percent Calories from Fat:* 22

DINNER
SPAGHETTI AND MEAT SAUCE*

1 cup green beans, steamed
Powdered butter substitute, such as Butter Buds or Molly
   McButter
   GARLIC BREAD*
Lettuce and tomato salad
2 tablespoons nonfat Italian dressing
¼ honeydew melon
½ cup orange sherbet

> *Total Calories:* 775
> *Grams of Fat:* 20.5
> *Percent Calories from Fat:* 24

DAY 4

BREAKFAST
HOT APPLE OATMEAL*
2 ounces Entenmann's "Fat Free" sweet roll, warmed
Regular/decaf coffee or tea with Nutrasweet, 1% low-fat milk
> *Total Calories: 585*
> *Grams of Fat: 4*
> *Percent Calories from Fat: 6*

LUNCH
CHICKEN SANDWICH
3 ounces skinless chicken breast (presliced, if desired)
1 tablespoon nonfat mayonnaise
1 teaspoon noncreamy mustard
Lettuce and tomato
2 slices cracked-wheat bread

Raw Vegetable Salad (see Day 2 dinner)
1 fresh pear
4 RyKrisp crackers, unseasoned
> *Total Calories: 506*
> *Grams of Fat: 6*
> *Percent Calories from Fat: 11*

DINNER
STEAK AND ONIONS*
¼ cup low-fat gravy
2 dinner rolls, heated
2 teaspoons Heart Beat margarine
Raw Vegetable Salad (see Day 2 dinner)
1 cup fresh or frozen strawberries (no sugar added)
½ cup peach sorbet, such as Dole
> *Total Calories: 744*
> *Grams of Fat: 15*
> *Percent Calories from Fat: 18*

DAY 5

FRENCH TOAST*

⅛ honeydew melon
Regular or decaf coffee, or tea with Nutrasweet, 1% low-fat
 milk
 Total Calories: 437
 Grams of Fat: 10
 Percent Calories from Fat: 21

LUNCH

TOASTED CHEESE AND TOMATO SANDWICH

2 slices cracked-wheat bread, toasted
3 slices nonfat presliced cheese, melted on toast
2 slices tomato, or to taste

1 orange
16 Wheat Thin crackers
 Total Calories: 500
 Grams of Fat: 8
 Percent Calories from Fat: 14

DINNER

CHILE AND CORN BREAD

Combine:
1 pound lean ground turkey, browned in nonstick vegetable
 spray
2 cans chile beans (no meat added)

1 4-inch square corn bread (made from mix)
2 teaspoons Heart Beat margarine
Raw Vegetable Salad (see Day 2 dinner)
1 fresh pear, quartered
½ cup instant pudding made with 1% low-fat milk
 Total Calories: 695
 Grams of Fat: 12
 Percent Calories from Fat: 16

DAY 6

BREAKFAST
QUICK BREAKFAST

3 ¾-ounce wedges Laughing Cow reduced-calorie cheese
2 apples, quartered
16 Oat Thin crackers
Regular/decaf coffee or tea with Nutrasweet, 1% low-fat milk

Total Calories: 365
Grams of Fat: 12
Percent Calories from Fat: 30

LUNCH
TURKEY AND CHEESE SANDWICH

2 1-ounce slices deli presliced turkey
1 slice nonfat presliced cheese
1 tablespoon nonfat mayonnaise
Lettuce and sliced tomato
2 slices 100% whole-wheat bread

10 Wheatsworth crackers
1 banana

Total Calories: 527
Grams of Fat: 10
Percent Calories from Fat: 17

DINNER
QUICK STIR-FRY*

1 fresh orange
2 ounces Entenmann's fat-free chocolate cake

Total Calories: 700
Grams of Fat: 13
Percent Calories from Fat: 17

DAY
7

BREAKFAST

PORTABLE BREAKFAST*
Total Calories: 490
Grams of Fat: 4
Percent Calories from Fat: 7

LUNCH

BLT SANDWICH
4 strips turkey bacon, cooked crisp with nonstick vegetable
   spray
Lettuce
2–3 thick slices tomato
2 tablespoons nonfat mayonnaise
2 slices Wonder Light white bread, toasted

1 fresh green apple, quartered
12 Harvest Crisp oat crackers
   Total Calories: 384
   Grams of Fat: 13
   Percent Calories from Fat: 30

DINNER

CHUCK ROAST*
1 slice sourdough bread
1 teaspoon Heart Beat margarine
½ banana, sliced crosswise
1 cup sugar-free Jell-O, or
½ cup custard made with 1% low-fat milk and Egg Beaters
   Total Calories: 742
   Grams of Fat: 15
   Percent Calories from Fat: 18

DAY 8

QUICKEST BREAKFAST

1 cup 1% low-fat milk
1 packet Carnation Instant Breakfast with Nutrasweet (any flavor)
2 slices 100% whole-grain bread, toasted
2 teaspoons Heart Beat margarine
2 teaspoons sugar-free jelly
1 banana
> *Total Calories:* 448
> *Grams of Fat:* 7
> *Percent Calories from Fat:* 14

LUNCH
EGG SALAD SANDWICH

Combine:
3 hard-boiled eggs, yolks removed from 2, diced
2 tablespoons nonfat mayonnaise
Noncreamy mustard
1 tablespoon pickle relish, or to taste
1/4 cup or more chopped celery

2 slices Branola bread
Lettuce and sliced tomato

16 Wheat Thins
1 peach
> *Total Calories:* 485
> *Grams of Fat:* 6
> *Percent Calories from Fat:* 11

DINNER
PORK AND BEANS

Combine:
1 pound extra-lean ground beef (no more than 15% fat), browned
2 16-ounce cans pork and beans with pork removed, heated

1 ear corn, boiled
Powdered butter substitute
Lettuce and tomato salad
2 tablespoons fat-free dressing
1 slice watermelon
2 Entenmann's fat-free oatmeal cookies
> *1 portion equals total of beef and beans*
> *Total Calories:* 719
> *Grams of Fat:* 11
> *Percent Calories from Fat:* 14

DAY 9

BREAKFAST
FAST BREAKFAST

1 6-ounce carton nonfat yogurt (with Nutrasweet)
1¼ cups fresh or frozen strawberries (no sugar added)
1 whole-grain English muffin (2 slices), toasted
4 teaspoons Heart Beat margarine
4 teaspoons honey
Regular or decaf coffee or tea with Nutrasweet, 1% low-fat milk

Total Calories: 417
Grams of Fat: 6
Percent Calories from Fat: 13

LUNCH
FRESH FRUIT AND COTTAGE CHEESE PLATE

1½ cups nonfat cottage cheese
1 cup your choice mixed fresh fruit (such as cantaloupe and honeydew balls)
16 Oat Thin crackers

Total Calories: 485
Grams of Fat: 6
Percent Calories from Fat: 11

DINNER
QUICK PIZZA*

½ cup nonfat frozen dairy dessert, such as Simple Pleasures

Total Calories: 780
Grams of Fat: 14
Percent Calories from Fat: 16

DAY 10

BREAKFAST
MUFFIN SANDWICH*
½ fresh grapefruit
Regular/decaf coffee or tea with Nutrasweet, 1% low-fat milk
Total Calories: 435
Grams of Fat: 12
Percent Calories from Fat: 25

LUNCH
CHEF SALAD*
1 fresh, Golden Delicious apple
Total Calories: 581
Grams of Fat: 7
Percent Calories from Fat: 12

DINNER
BEEF STEW*
2 slices sourdough bread
2 teaspoons Heart Beat margarine
¼ cantaloupe
½ cup nonfat frozen yogurt
Total Calories: 830
Grams of Fat: 14
Percent Calories from Fat: 15

DAY 11

BREAKFAST

EGG BURRITO*

1 medium-size peach, halved
1 cup 1% low-fat milk
Regular/decaf coffee or tea with Nutrasweet, 1% low-fat milk
Total Calories: 422
Grams of Fat: 8
Percent Calories from Fat: 17

LUNCH

WHOLE-WHEAT PITA SANDWICH

2 slices lean deli beef, presliced
2 slices nonfat presliced cheese
2 tablespoons nonfat mayonnaise
lettuce to taste
1 whole-wheat pita, sliced down middle to form 2 semicircles
10 premium whole-wheat saltines
1 cup watermelon balls
Total Calories: 449
Grams of Fat: 7
Percent Calories from Fat: 14

DINNER

HEALTHY, HEARTY HAMBURGERS

1 3-ounce (cooked weight) extra-lean ground beef patty (no more than 15% fat), broiled
2 tablespoons nonfat mayonnaise
Mustard, ketchup, relish
Lettuce, tomato
1 whole-wheat bun, such as Roman Meal, toasted
½ cup Heinz beans in tomato sauce
1 fresh apple, quartered
BANANA SPLIT
4 ounces nonfat ice cream
½ banana, sliced
1 tablespoon Hershey's chocolate syrup (it has no fat) (optional)
Total Calories: 789
Grams of Fat: 16
Percent Calories from Fat: 18

DAY 12

BONUS BREAKFAST

1 egg, scrambled in nonstick vegetable spray (mixed with 1 tablespoon 1% low-fat milk, if desired)
1 whole bagel (2 slices), toasted
2 tablespoons "light" Philadelphia Cream Cheese
2 tablespoons sugar-free jelly

OATMEAL

Combine:
½ cup cooked oatmeal (or about 2½ tablespoons uncooked, using ½ cup water)
2 tablespoons raisins, added while cooking
½ cup 1% low-fat milk, added after cooking
Regular/decaf coffee or tea with Nutrasweet, 1% low-fat milk

Total Calories: 480
Grams of Fat: 16
Percent Calories from Fat: 30

BRAWNY BURRITO*

½ cup Van Camp's canned Spanish rice, heated

FRUIT SALAD

1 kiwi fruit, sliced
½ cup fresh or frozen strawberries (no sugar added)

Total Calories: 555
Grams of Fat: 16
Percent Calories from Fat: 26

BROILED RED SNAPPER WITH TARTAR SAUCE

6 ounces red snapper, broiled

TARTAR SAUCE

1 tablespoon fat-free mayonnaise
2 teaspoons pickle relish
⅛ teaspoon lemon juice (or substitute by itself for tartar sauce)
Pinch of dried parsley

1 large potato, baked
1 cup broccoli, steamed
Lettuce and tomato salad
2 tablespoons nonfat dressing
1 whole-wheat dinner roll
1 teaspoon Heart Beat margarine
½ cup lime sherbet

Total Calories: 748
Grams of Fat: 7
Percent Calories from Fat: 8

DAY 13

BREAKFAST BURGER

1 1½-ounce extra-lean beef (no more than 15% fat) patty, broiled

1 slice nonfat American cheese

2 teaspoons Heart Beat margarine, or 2 tablespoons nonfat mayonnaise

1 English muffin (2 slices), toasted

1 cup fresh or frozen blueberries (no sugar added)

8 ounces 1% low-fat milk (beverage)

Regular/decaf coffee or tea with Nutrasweet, 1% low-fat milk

Total Calories: 447

Grams of Fat: 12.5

Percent Calories from Fat: 25

HEARTY SOUP

10¾ ounces Campbell's "Chunky" vegetable beef soup

18 5-gram Harvest crackers

1 fresh apple

Total Calories: 430

Grams of Fat: 11

Percent Calories from Fat: 23

CHICKEN FAJITAS*

⅔ cup rice (Minute rice or steamed)

Powdered butter substitute, such as Molly McButter

1 cup zucchini cubes, steamed

⅛ honeydew melon

½ cup orange sherbet

Total Calories: 801

Grams of Fat: 10

Percent Calories from Fat: 11

DAY 14

BREAKFAST
FRUIT AND COTTAGE CHEESE SALAD
1 cup nonfat cottage cheese
1 ½ cups fruit medley, your choice of fruits

2 slices pumpernickel bread, toasted
2 teaspoons Heart Beat margarine
2 teaspoons sugar-free jelly or marmalade
Regular/decaf coffee or tea with Nutrasweet, 1% low-fat milk
> *Total Calories:* 420
> *Grams of Fat:* 4
> *Percent Calories from Fat:* 9

LUNCH
CLUB SANDWICH
2 ounces skinless presliced deli turkey
2 strips turkey bacon, browned with nonstick vegetable spray
Lettuce and sliced tomato
2 tablespoons nonfat mayonnaise
2 slices multigrain bread, toasted
> *Total Calories:* 434
> *Grams of Fat:* 9
> *Percent Calories from Fat:* 19

DINNER
BRAWNY BURRITO*
½ cup Van Camp's canned Spanish rice
Lemon juice to taste (for rice)
1 orange, sliced
½ cup instant vanilla pudding made with 1% low-fat milk
> *Total Calories:* 710
> *Grams of Fat:* 16
> *Percent Calories from Fat:* 20

DAY 15

BREAKFAST
VEGETABLE OMELETTE*
2 slices oat-bran bread, toasted
2 teaspoons Heart Beat margarine
2 teaspoons sugar-free jelly
1 fresh orange, cut into slices
Regular/decaf coffee or tea with Nutrasweet, 1% low-fat milk
> *Total Calories:* 465
> *Grams of Fat:* 10
> *Percent Calories from Fat:* 19

LUNCH
TIME-SAVER SOUP
10¾ ounces Campbell's Thick and Chunky chicken-rice soup
2 teaspoons Heart Beat margarine
2 slices whole-wheat bread
1 fresh pear
> *Total Calories:* 370
> *Grams of Fat:* 10
> *Percent Calories from Fat:* 24

DINNER
GUILT-FREE LASAGNA
2 cups of your favorite lasagna recipe, made with extra-lean ground beef (no more than 15% fat), nonfat cottage cheese instead of ricotta, and Lifetime low-fat mozzarella
1 cup French-cut green beans, steamed
GARLIC BREAD*
2 ounces Entenmann's fat-free orange pound cake
> *Total Calories:* 754
> *Grams of Fat:* 16
> *Percent Calories from Fat:* 19

DAY 16

FAST ORANGE LIFT*
2 slices seven-grain bread, toasted
2 teaspoons Heart Beat margarine
2 teaspoons sugar-free jelly
Regular/decaf coffee or tea with Nutrasweet, 1% low-fat milk
Total Calories: 418
Grams of Fat: 6
Percent Calories from Fat: 13

LUNCH
CRAB SALAD
Combine:
6 ounces frozen or canned cooked crab
2 tablespoons nonfat mayonnaise
Bed of lettuce

10¾ ounces Campbell's New England clam chowder
2 slices French bread
2 teaspoons Heart Beat margarine
½ cup fresh pineapple chunks
Total Calories: 424
Grams of Fat: 11
Percent Calories from Fat: 23

DINNER
STEAK AND SHRIMP PLATTER
3½ ounces lean tenderloin steak (fat trimmed), broiled
6 large shrimp, broiled
Powdered butter substitute (or lemon juice) for shrimp
1 large potato, baked
2 tablespoons nonfat sour cream
1 cup broccoli, steamed
Lettuce and tomato salad
2 tablespoons nonfat dressing
1 cup fresh or frozen strawberries (no sugar added)
1 cup rice custard made with 1% low-fat milk and Egg Beaters
Total Calories: 689
Grams of Fat: 11
Percent Calories from Fat: 14

DAY 17

BREAKFAST

LO-CAL OMELETTE*
1 whole English muffin (2 slices), toasted
2 teaspoons Heart Beat margarine
2 teaspoons sugar-free jelly
Regular/decaf coffee or tea with Nutrasweet, 1% low-fat milk
Total Calories: 430
Grams of Fat: 4
Percent Calories from Fat: 8

LUNCH

SALMON SALAD SANDWICH
Combine:
4 ounces (½ can) canned salmon
2 tablespoons nonfat mayonnaise
Pickle, relish, celery, and onions, as desired, chopped
2 slices 100% whole-wheat bread

Lettuce and tomato salad
2 tablespoons nonfat Ranch dressing
½ banana
4 RyKrisp crackers
Total Calories: 550
Grams of Fat: 10
Percent Calories from Fat: 16

DINNER

LOBSTER PLATE
6-ounce lobster, broiled or steamed
Lemon to taste (add to butter substitute for lobster)
1 potato, baked
POTATO FILLING
Blend:
¼ cup nonfat cottage cheese
Chives to taste
Powdered butter substitute (save some for lobster)

1 cup asparagus, steamed
1 slice sourdough bread
¼ cantaloupe
½ cup nonfat dairy dessert, such as Simple Pleasures
Total Calories: 741
Grams of Fat: 3
Percent Calories from Fat: 4

DAY 18

BREAKFAST
MEXICAN OMELETTE*
Regular/decaf coffee or tea with Nutrasweet, 1% low-fat milk
> *Total Calories:* 450
> *Grams of Fat:* 10
> *Percent Calories from Fat:* 20

LUNCH
SPINACH SALAD
Combine:
2 cups chopped fresh spinach
3 hard-boiled eggs, yolks removed from 2, chopped
2 strips turkey bacon cooked in nonfat vegetable spray, diced

2 tablespoons nonfat vinaigrette dressing

8 Wheat Thin crackers
FRUIT SALAD
1 fresh orange, chopped
1 banana, sliced crosswise
> *Total Calories:* 550
> *Grams of Fat:* 10
> *Percent Calories from Fat:* 16

DINNER
VEGETABLE BEEF SOUP*
2 slices pumpernickel bread
2 teaspoons Heart Beat margarine
1 fresh peach, sliced
½ cup raspberry sorbet
> *Total Calories:* 635
> *Grams of Fat:* 15
> *Percent Calories from Fat:* 21

DAY 19

BREAKFAST
PEANUT BUTTER AND JELLY JUMP START
2 tablespoons Laura Scudder's old-fashioned natural peanut butter
2 teaspoons sugar-free jelly
2 slices multigrain bread
⅓ cup cooked oatmeal
½ cup 1% low-fat milk (for oatmeal)
2 fresh apricots
Regular/decaf coffee or tea with Nutrasweet, 1% low-fat milk
NOTE: For an *occasional* reward make peanut butter and jelly sandwich and serve with cooked oatmeal and apricots.
> *Total Calories: 465*
> *Grams of Fat: 19*
> *Percent Calories from Fat: 37*

LUNCH
LEAN PATTIMELT*
Lettuce and tomato salad
2 tablespoons nonfat blue cheese dressing
2 cups honeydew or cantaloupe balls
> *Total Calories: 477*
> *Grams of Fat: 12*
> *Percent Calories from Fat: 23*

DINNER
STEAK SANDWICH
Chopped onion and tomato, sautéed in nonstick vegetable oil
3½ ounces lean tenderloin (fat trimmed), broiled
Ketchup and mustard to taste
1 6-inch French roll, toasted

Lettuce and tomato salad (large)
1 cup fresh pineapple chunks
ROOT BEER FLOAT
½ cup nonfat vanilla ice cream, such as Simple Pleasures
Diet root beer
> *Total Calories: 601*
> *Grams of Fat: 11*
> *Percent Calories from Fat: 17*

DAY 20

BREAKFAST
HOT CEREAL AND BACON*
1 slice 100% whole-wheat bread, toasted
1 teaspoon Heart Beat margarine
1 teaspoon sugar-free jelly
Regular/decaf coffee or tea with Nutrasweet, 1% low-fat milk
> *Total Calories: 458*
> *Grams of Fat: 7*
> *Percent Calories from Fat: 14*

LUNCH
TURKEY AND SWISS SANDWICH
2 1-ounce slices smoked turkey
1 slice nonfat presliced Swiss cheese
1 tablespoon nonfat Miracle Whip dressing
Lettuce and sliced tomato
2 slices sourdough bread
CARROT RAISIN SALAD
1 cup shredded carrot
2 tablespoons raisins
2 tablespoons nonfat mayonnaise
1 package Nutrasweet
A few drops of vinegar

½ cup fresh pineapple chunks
> *Total Calories: 439*
> *Grams of Fat: 4*
> *Percent Calories from Fat: 8*

DINNER
SLOPPY JOE*
1 cup mashed potatoes made with 1% low-fat milk and butter substitute
½ cup corn niblets, heated
Lettuce and tomato salad
2 tablespoons nonfat dressing
¼ cup banana, sliced crosswise
¼ cup orange slices
½ cup raspberry sorbet
> *Total Calories: 780*
> *Grams of Fat: 16*
> *Percent Calories from Fat: 19*

DAY 21

BREAKFAST

HAM AND HOME FRIES*

1 slice sourdough bread, toasted
1 teaspoon diet Heart Beat margarine
1 teaspoon sugar-free jelly
1/4 cantaloupe
Regular/decaf coffee or tea with Nutrasweet, 1% low-fat milk

Total Calories: 353
Grams of Fat: 10
Percent Calories from Fat: 25

LUNCH

LEAN HOAGIE

1 slice nonfat presliced Swiss cheese
1 slice nonfat American cheese
1 1-ounce slice 98% fat-free presliced deli ham
1 1-ounce slice turkey salami, such as Louis Rich
1 1-ounce slice turkey pastrami
Lettuce, sliced tomato, and sliced onion
1 tablespoon nonfat mayonnaise
1 6-inch French roll, sliced
1 fresh pear

COLE SLAW

Combine:
1 cup shredded cabbage
1 cup shredded carrots
2 tablespoons nonfat mayonnaise
1 package Nutrasweet
A few drops of cider vinegar

Total Calories: 436
Grams of Fat: 6
Percent Calories from Fat: 12

DINNER

QUESADILLAS*

1/2 cup Van Camp's canned Spanish rice
Lettuce and tomato salad
Salsa (instead of salad dressing)
Lemon (for salad)
3 kiwi fruits, sliced
1/2 cup instant chocolate pudding made with 1% low-fat milk

Total Calories: 760
Grams of Fat: 8
Percent Calories from Fat: 9

DAY 22

BREAKFAST
HEARTY MORNING MEAL
3 4-inch buttermilk pancakes from Aunt Jemima frozen batter
Powdered butter substitute, such as Butter Buds
Sugar-free jelly or syrup (as topping)
1 whole egg and 2 egg whites, scrambled in nonstick vegetable spray with 1 tablespoon 1% low-fat milk (optional)
1 1-ounce slice 98% fat-free presliced deli ham, hot or cold
½ cup fresh or frozen orange juice
Regular/decaf coffee or tea with Nutrasweet, 1% low-fat milk
  Total Calories: 389
  Grams of Fat: 9
  Percent Calories from Fat: 21

LUNCH
CHICKEN SALAD PLATE
Combine:
3 ounces canned white meat chicken
2 tablespoons nonfat mayonnaise
1 tablespoon chopped celery
1 tablespoon pickle relish
1 tablespoon chopped onion, if desired
Shredded lettuce

4 RyKrisp crackers
  Total Calories: 529
  Grams of Fat: 6
  Percent Calories from Fat: 10

DINNER
SOFT TACOS*
½ cup Van Camp's canned Spanish rice
Diced tomato, onion, and lettuce (as garnish)
2 fresh tangerines
½ cup nonfat ice cream
  Total Calories: 760
  Grams of Fat: 18
  Percent Calories from Fat: 21

DAY 23

BREAKFAST
WAFFLES AND EGGS
2 Eggo Nutri-Grain waffles
Butter Buds liquid butter substitute
2 tablespoons sugar-free strawberry jelly
1 whole egg and 2 egg whites, scrambled in nonstick vegetable spray

⅛ honeydew melon
Regular/decaf coffee or tea with Nutrasweet, 1% low-fat milk
Total Calories: 472
Grams of Fat: 16
Percent Calories from Fat: 31

LUNCH
TUNA PITA
Combine:
1 6⅛-ounce can water-packed tuna
1 tablespoon each chopped celery, pickle relish, or chopped onion
2 tablespoons nonfat mayonnaise
1 whole-wheat pita, cut to form 2 semicircles

8 Ritz crackers
1 fresh peach
Total Calories: 514
Grams of Fat: 12
Percent Calories from Fat: 21

DINNER
SWEDISH MEATBALLS*
1 cup fresh French-cut green beans, steamed
2 1-inch-thick slices French bread
2 teaspoons Heart Beat margarine
4 fresh apricots
½ cup rainbow sherbet
Total Calories: 770
Grams of Fat: 19
Percent Calories from Fat: 22

DAY 24

BREAKFAST
STRAWBERRIES AND YOGURT

1¼ cups fresh or frozen strawberries (no sugar added)
1 cup plain or vanilla Yoplait yogurt
2 slices oat-bran bread, toasted
2 teaspoons Heart Beat margarine
2 teaspoons sugar-free jelly
2 slices (about 2 ounces) Canadian bacon, crisped using nonstick vegetable spray
Regular/decaf coffee or tea with Nutrasweet, 1% low-fat milk
  Total Calories: 410
  Grams of Fat: 6
  Percent Calories from Fat: 13

LUNCH
ROAST BEEF ON SOURDOUGH SANDWICH

2 2-ounce slices Swiss cheese
3 1-ounce slices 98% fat-free presliced deli beef
1 tablespoon nonfat Miracle Whip dressing
Noncreamy mustard and pickle chips
Sliced onion and jalapeño pepper, if desired
Tomato slices
2 slices sourdough bread

Cole Slaw (see Day 21 lunch)
1 cup fresh or frozen raspberries (no sugar added)
  Total Calories: 409
  Grams of Fat: 5
  Percent Calories from Fat: 11

DINNER
BAKED HAM DELUXE

3 ounces lean (at least 96% fat-free) prebaked ham
½ cup mashed potatoes made with 1% low-fat milk and butter substitute
½ cup canned yams, heated
1 cup Brussels sprouts, steamed
2 dinner rolls, heated
2 teaspoons Heart Beat margarine
1 cup fresh or frozen raspberries (no sugar added)
½ cup sliced peaches
½ cup nonfat vanilla ice cream
  Total Calories: 715
  Grams of Fat: 8
  Percent Calories from Fat: 10

DAY 25

BREAKFAST
APPLE SPUDS AND HAM*
2 slices rye bread, toasted
2 teaspoons Heart Beat margarine
2 teaspoons sugar-free jelly
Regular/decaf coffee or tea with Nutrasweet, 1% low-fat milk
> *Total Calories: 410*
> *Grams of Fat: 6*
> *Percent Calories from Fat: 13*

LUNCH
CHEESE AND CRACKERS
22 Wheat Thin Crackers
2 ounces Lifetime cheese (comes in brick form), sliced
1 large carrot, cut into sticks
2 celery stalks, cut into sticks
2 tablespoons nonfat Ranch dressing (dip for carrot and celery)
FRUIT SALAD
1 banana, sliced crosswise
1 orange, sliced
> *Total Calories: 581*
> *Grams of Fat: 18*
> *Percent Calories from Fat: 28*

DINNER
CHUCK WAGON STEAK
1 3-ounce extra-lean (no more than 15% fat) ground beef patty, browned in skillet
1 cup mashed potatoes made with 1% low-fat milk and butter substitute
Cauliflower and broccoli, steamed
2 whole-grain dinner rolls
1 cup fresh or frozen blueberries (no sugar added)
½ cup nonfat pistachio frozen yogurt
> *Total Calories: 733*
> *Grams of Fat: 17*
> *Percent Calories from Fat: 21*

DAY 26

BREAKFAST
BANANA YOGURT
Combine:
1 banana, sliced crosswise
1 6-ounce carton nonfat vanilla yogurt (with Nutrasweet)

2 slices 100% whole-wheat bread, toasted
2 teaspoons Heart Beat margarine
2 teaspoons sugar-free jelly
Regular/decaf coffee or tea with Nutrasweet, 1% low-fat milk
> *Total Calories:* 380
> *Grams of Fat:* 5
> *Percent Calories from Fat:* 12

LUNCH
TOASTED TURKEY OR HAM AND CHEESE SANDWICH
4 slices turkey pastrami
1 slice nonfat Swiss or American presliced cheese, melted on toast
Noncreamy mustard
1–2 slices tomato
Lettuce and pickle chips
2 slices rye bread, toasted
FRUIT-SPICE YOGURT
Combine:
3 tablespoons raisins
1 apple, diced
¼ teaspoon cinnamon
1 6-ounce carton nonfat vanilla yogurt (with Nutrasweet)
> *Total Calories:* 490
> *Grams of Fat:* 4
> *Percent Calories from Fat:* 7

DINNER
LEAN MEAT LOAF*
1 cup mashed potatoes made with 1% low-fat milk and butter substitute
½ cup fresh peas, and 1 cup carrots, steamed
2 slices sourdough bread
2 teaspoons Heart Beat margarine (for bread)
3 fresh plums
½ cup instant tapioca pudding made with 1% low-fat milk
> *Total Calories:* 775
> *Grams of Fat:* 21
> *Percent Calories from fat:* 18

DAY 27

BREAKFAST

HAM AND SWISS OMELETTE*
1 whole-wheat bagel (2 slices), toasted
2 teaspoons Heart Beat margarine
2 teaspoons sugar-free jelly
½ cup fresh pineapple chunks
Regular/decaf coffee or tea with Nutrasweet, 1% low-fat milk
> *Total Calories:* 390
> *Grams of Fat:* 12
> *Percent Calories from Fat:* 28

LUNCH

TURKEY PASTRAMI ON RYE
4 1-ounce slices Louis Rich turkey pastrami
Noncreamy mustard
2 tablespoons nonfat mayonnaise, if desired
Tomato, lettuce, diced onion, and pickle chips
2 slices whole rye bread
½ cup thinly sliced cucumber
Lettuce
Tomato (optional)
1 tablespoon nonfat French dressing
2 bread sticks
6 fresh apricots
> *Total Calories:* 459
> *Grams of Fat:* 6
> *Percent Calories from Fat:* 11.8

DINNER

BEEF, CHEESE, AND NOODLE CASSEROLE*
1 cup fresh spinach, steamed
Powdered butter substitute (for spinach, if topping is desired)
2 whole-wheat dinner rolls, heated
2 teaspoons Heart Beat margarine
Lettuce and tomato salad
2 tablespoons nonfat dressing
1 cup fresh grapefruit
½ cup nonfat rum raisin ice cream
> *Total Calories:* 737
> *Grams of Fat:* 14
> *Percent Calories from Fat:* 17

DAY 28

BREAKFAST
HOT CEREAL AND BAGEL
3 tablespoons Malt-O-Meal (cooking instructions on box)
½ cup 1% low-fat milk
1 tablespoon honey
1 1-ounce slice 98% fat-free presliced deli ham
1 whole oat-bran bagel (2 slices), toasted
2 teaspoons Heart Beat margarine
2 teaspoons sugar-free jelly
Regular/decaf coffee or tea with Nutrasweet, 1% low-fat milk
> *Total Calories:* 470
> *Grams of Fat:* 6
> *Percent Calories from Fat:* 11

LUNCH
TOASTED TUNA MELT
Combine:
3 ounces (½ can) water-packed tuna
2 tablespoons nonfat mayonnaise
Diced celery
1 tablespoon pickle relish
2 slices 100% whole-wheat bread, toasted
1 slice nonfat American cheese, melted on toast
> *Total Calories:* 464
> *Grams of Fat:* 4
> *Percent Calories from Fat:* 8

DINNER
HAM AND BEANS
3 ounces lean prebaked ham (at least 96% fat-free), heated
   or fried in nonstick vegetable spray
½ cup Heinz beans in tomato sauce
1 cup steamed or boiled rice
Raw Vegetable Salad (see Day 2 dinner)
2 tablespoons nonfat dressing
½ 6-inch French bread roll
1 teaspoon Heart Beat margarine
1 cup fresh or frozen strawberries
½ cup nonfat vanilla ice cream
> *Total Calories:* 755
> *Grams of Fat:* 7
> *Percent Calories from Fat:* 8

DAY 29

ENGLISH BREAKFAST

1 egg, cooked over-easy with nonstick vegetable spray
2 strips turkey bacon, crisped with nonstick vegetable spray
1 whole English muffin (2 slices), toasted
2 teaspoons Heart Beat margarine
2 teaspoons sugar-free jelly
1 fresh apple, quartered
Regular/decaf coffee or tea with Nutrasweet, 1% low-fat milk
  Total Calories: 350
  Grams of Fat: 14
  Percent Calories from Fat: 36

HAM AND CHEESE ON PUMPERNICKEL

2 1-ounce slices 98% fat-free presliced deli ham
1 slice nonfat Alpine Lace Swiss cheese
2 tablespoons nonfat mayonnaise
2 slices pumpernickel bread

16 Wheat Thins crackers
1 cup (about 20) fresh Bing cherries
  Total Calories: 519
  Grams of Fat: 10
  Percent Calories from Fat: 17

BEEF STROGANOFF*

Green salad
2 tablespoons nonfat dressing
1 dinner roll, heated
1 teaspoon Heart Beat margarine
½ cup nonfat strawberries and cream frozen yogurt
  Total Calories: 828
  Grams of Fat: 14
  Percent Calories from Fat: 15

DAY 30

BREAKFAST
SCRAMBLED EGGS IN TORTILLAS*
1¼ cups watermelon balls
Regular/decaf coffee or tea with Nutrasweet, 1% low-fat milk
> *Total Calories:* 407
> *Grams of Fat:* 9
> *Percent Calories from Fat:* 22

LUNCH
HEALTHY HOT DOGS
2 90% fat-free Hormel hot dogs (under 5 grams fat per hot dog)
Mustard, ketchup, relish, and onion
2 whole-grain hot dog buns

½ cup pork and beans with pork fat removed
Lettuce and tomato salad
1 tablespoon nonfat dressing
1 slice watermelon
> *Total Calories:* 514
> *Grams of Fat:* 14
> *Percent Calories from Fat:* 24.5

DINNER
LEAN BACON CHEESEBURGER
1 2-ounce extra-lean (no more than 15% fat) beef patty, broiled
2 strips turkey bacon, crisped in nonstick vegetable spray
1 slice nonfat American cheese
Lettuce, tomato, onion, mustard, and ketchup to taste
1 tablespoon fat-free mayonnaise
1 whole-grain bun

½ cup corn niblets cooked
½ potato, cut into wedges, seasoned to taste, baked at 400° F. for 35–45 minutes (on pan sprayed with nonstick vegetable spray)
1 cup watermelon balls
1 ounce Entenmann's fat-free chocolate cake
> *Total Calories:* 735
> *Grams of Fat:* 15
> *Percent Calories from Fat:* 18

RECIPES, BY DAY

BREAKFAST

HAM AND CHEESE OMELETTE *(Day 1)*

> 1 1-ounce slice 98% fat-free presliced deli ham, chopped
> 1 whole egg and 2 egg whites, beaten together
> 1 slice nonfat presliced cheese, such as Kraft

Mix chopped ham with beaten eggs and pour into an omelette pan coated with nonstick vegetable spray; when one side is done, add cheese slice and flip the omelette over to complete.

SCRAMBLED EGGS *(Day 2)*

> 1 whole egg and 2 egg whites
> 1 tablespoon 1% low-fat milk (optional)
> 1 medium-size potato, baked or boiled the night before,
>   cut crosswise into ⅛-inch slices

Beat eggs and add milk, if desired. Cook beaten eggs in skillet coated with nonstick vegetable spray. In another skillet coated with nonstick vegetable spray, fry potato slices until golden brown.

HOT APPLE OATMEAL *(Day 4)*

> 1 cup raw oats
> ¼ cup peeled, diced apple
> 2 tablespoons raisins
> 2 teaspoons brown sugar, molasses, or Nutrasweet
> ⅛ teaspoon cinnamon
> 1 cup 1% low-fat milk

Before cooking oats, add apple chunks; raisins; cinnamon; and brown sugar, molasses, or Nutrasweet. Cook oats according to package instructions. Add milk when the oatmeal has finished cooking.

FRENCH TOAST *(Day 5)*

> 1 whole egg and 2 egg whites, beaten together
> 1 teaspoon vanilla extract
> ⅛ teaspoon cinnamon
> 2 tablespoons 1% low-fat milk
> 2 slices 100% whole-wheat bread
> Powdered butter substitute, such as Butter Buds
> 2 tablespoons sugar-free jelly, or 2 tablespoons regular syrup
> 1 slice (about 1 ounce) Canadian bacon

Mix egg and egg whites with vanilla extract, cinnamon, and milk. Dip bread into mixture, making sure to coat each slice thoroughly. Fry in skillet sprayed with nonstick vegetable spray, and cook any leftover batter into scrambled eggs. Top French toast with the butter substitute and jelly or syrup. Be sure to use vegetable spray on pan when you crisp the Canadian bacon, too.

PORTABLE BREAKFAST *(Day 7)*

> 1½ cups 1% low-fat milk
> 1 banana
> 1 6-ounce carton nonfat strawberry yogurt (with Nutrasweet)
> 1 tablespoon wheat germ
> 1 tablespoon vanilla-flavored 90% protein powder, or ¼ cup Egg Beaters

Add all ingredients together in a blender and mix to make the perfect portable breakfast.

MUFFIN SANDWICH *(Day 10)*

> *1 egg*
> *2 1-ounce slices 98% fat-free presliced deli ham*
> *1 whole-grain English muffin (2 slices)*
> *2 slices nonfat presliced cheese*
> *2 teaspoons Heart Beat margarine*

Fry the egg on both sides in skillet sprayed with nonstick vegetable spray. You can fry the ham the same way, heat it in the microwave, or serve it cool. Place the egg on top of one muffin slice, then top with ham and cheese. Spread margarine over the other muffin half before closing the sandwich. (You can melt your cheese in the microwave, if desired).

EGG BURRITO *(Day 11)*

> *1 whole egg and 2 egg whites*
> *1 tablespoon 1% low-fat milk (optional)*
> *2 slices nonfat presliced cheese, chopped*
> *2 6-inch or 1 12-inch whole-wheat tortilla*
> *¼ cup salsa*

Beat egg and egg whites and add milk if desired. Scramble eggs in a skillet coated with nonstick vegetable spray. As you cook the eggs, add cheese pieces, making sure they melt. Put eggs on tortilla, which you can heat beforehand in the microwave.

VEGETABLE OMELETTE *(Day 15)*

> *1 whole egg and 2 egg whites, beaten together*
> *Diced onion, tomato, bell pepper, parsley, sprouts to*
> *   taste*
> *2 slices nonfat presliced cheese*

Mix the egg and egg whites with the chopped onion, tomato, bell pepper, parsley, and sprouts. Then pour into omelette pan coated with nonstick vegetable spray and cook, adding cheese slice just after flipping.

FAST ORANGE LIFT *(Day 16)*

> *1 cup 1% low-fat milk*
> *1 cup fresh or frozen orange juice*
> *2 teaspoons vanilla extract*
> *½ cup Egg Beaters egg substitute*
> *6–8 ice cubes*
> *4–6 packages (1 teaspoon each) Nutrasweet*

Add all ingredients to blender carafe and blend on high until frothy.

LO-CAL OMELETTE *(Day 17)*

> *1 cup Egg Beaters egg substitute*
> *Diced onion and tomato to taste*
> *2 slices nonfat Alpine Lace Swiss cheese*

Mix together Egg Beaters and tomato-and-onion bits (your choice of onion, though white onion works well); be sure to coat omelette pan with nonstick vegetable spray before cooking. Cheese is added after flipping omelette.

MEXICAN OMELETTE *(Day 18)*

> *1 whole egg and 2 egg whites, beaten together*
> *¼ cup salsa*
> *1 once nonfat presliced American cheese*

> *½ cup Rosarita vegetarian refried beans*
> *2 6-inch whole-wheat or white flour tortillas, warmed*
> *½ cup fresh pineapple chunks*

Add salsa and cheese to beaten egg and egg whites. Cook in skillet sprayed with nonstick vegetable spray.

Heat the refried beans, wrap them in warmed tortillas, and serve with omelette and pineapple chunks.

HOT CEREAL AND BACON *(Day 20)*

> *2 slices (about 2 ounces) Canadian bacon*
> *1 cup cooked-wheat cereal, such as Cream of Wheat or Wheatena*
> *1 tablespoon raisins*
> *½ cup 1% low-fat milk*
> *1 tablespoon brown sugar*

Use nonstick vegetable spray when crisping bacon. Cook the cereal and mix the raisins, milk, and brown sugar into your cereal once it's done.

HAM AND HOME FRIES *(Day 21)*

> *1 medium-size potato, baked or boiled night before, cut crosswise into ⅛-inch slices*
> *2 1-ounce slices 98% fat-free presliced deli ham*
> *1 egg, cooked over-easy*

Fry potato slices in pan coated with nonstick vegetable spray until slices turn golden brown or crispy. If you wish to heat your ham, either fry it (with vegetable spray) or heat it in the microwave. Serve potatoes and ham alongside egg.

APPLE SPUDS AND HAM *(Day 25)*

> 1 *medium-size potato, baked or boiled night before, cut crosswise into ⅛-inch slices*
> 2 *1-ounce slices 98% fat-free presliced deli ham, heated*
> 1 *cup cinnamon applesauce*

Fry potato in pan with nonstick vegetable spray until slices are golden. To heat the ham, either fry with nonstick vegetable spray or microwave. Serve potatoes and ham with applesauce.

HAM AND SWISS OMELETTE *(Day 29)*

> 1 *whole egg and 2 egg whites, beaten*
> 1 *ounce 98% fat-free presliced deli ham, chopped*
> 1 *ounce low-fat Swiss cheese (2 to 3 grams fat, max)*

Follow omelette instructions for Day 1 breakfast, substituting low-fat Swiss for nonfat cheese.

SCRAMBLED EGGS IN TORTILLAS *(Day 30)*

> 1 *whole egg and 2 egg whites, beaten*
> *Diced onion, tomato, and bell pepper to taste*
> 1 *1-ounce slice Louis Rich turkey pastrami, chopped*
> 2 *6-inch or 1 12-inch flour tortillas, warmed*

Scramble eggs in a skillet coated with nonstick vegetable spray, adding onion, tomato, bell pepper, and turkey pastrami as eggs cook. Cook till all ingredients are heated through. When done, wrap tortilla(s) around eggs.

LUNCH

CHEF SALAD *(Day 10)*

> 2 1-gram slices each of Hillshire Farms lean beef, ham,
>   and turkey
> 1 slice nonfat presliced cheese
> 2 hard-boiled eggs, yolks removed
> Lettuce
> Sliced cucumbers and tomatoes—as much as desired
> ¼ cup nonfat dressing
> 4 bread sticks

Cut meat and cheese into strips; egg whites are cubed. Place on bed of lettuce, along with cucumber and tomato slices, before pouring on dressing. You can add any other *raw* vegetables you desire to the salad as well. Serve with bread sticks.

BRAWNY BURRITO *(Day 12)*

> Taco sauce to taste
> 2 ounces extra-lean ground beef (no more than 15%
>   fat)
> ½ cup Rosarita vegetarian refried beans
> 1 12-inch wheat- or white-flour tortilla
> Diced tomato and onion to taste
> 2 tablespoons nonfat sour cream

Follow directions on the packet of taco seasoning to cook the beef. Heat the refried beans, following package directions as well. When the beef is ready, heat the tortilla in a microwave or oven, then fill with beef, adding tomato and onion bits as well as low-fat sour cream.

LEAN PATTIMELT *(Day 19)*

> *2 ounces extra-lean (no more than 15% fat) ground*
> *   round*
> *2 slices rye bread, toasted*
> *1 ounce nonfat Swiss cheese*

Form beef into patty, and brown in skillet. Top one slice of bread with it. Place cheese on the other slice, and microwave for 20 seconds, or broil, until cheese melts; add to patty.

DINNER

BARBECUED SHISH KEBAB *(Day 1)*

> *3½ ounces (per portion) lean top round*
> *¾ teaspoon chili powder*
> *¼ teaspoon garlic powder*
> *¼ teaspoon dried oregano*
> *⅛ teaspoon ground cumin*
> *Chunks of onion, zucchini, cherry tomato, celery, bell*
> *   peppers, mushroom to taste*

Cut beef into 1-square-inch cubes. Mix the seasonings with the beef, blending well to ensure that the seasoning is evenly distributed over chunks. Cover the bowl tightly and refrigerate up to 2 hours prior to cooking. Then place beef on skewers, alternating it with vegetable chunks. Cook on barbecue or on broiler, turning frequently, for 8 to 12 minutes, or until done.

SPAGHETTI AND MEAT SAUCE *(Day 3)*

> *1 pound extra-lean (no more than 15% fat) ground beef*
> *1 30-ounce jar spaghetti sauce of choice*
> *8 ounces dry spaghetti noodles, cooked following direc-*
> *   tions on package*

Brown the beef using nonstick vegetable spray, draining off any fat. Once beef is done, pour in the jar of spaghetti sauce. Simmer on low heat for 30 to 60 minutes before adding to the noodles.

GARLIC BREAD *(Day 3)*

> 2 1-inch-thick slices French bread
> 2 teaspoons Heart Beat margarine
> Garlic powder to taste

To make garlic bread, simply spread margarine over bread slices, sprinkle with garlic powder and toast.

STEAK AND ONIONS *(Day 4)*

> 3 ounces lean flank steak, fat trimmed
> 1 small onion, sliced
> 1 medium potato, cut into thirds
> 2 carrots, skinned and sliced

Season steak to taste and wrap in aluminum foil along with onion, potato slices, and carrots. Bake for 2 to 2½ hours at 325° F.

QUICK STIR-FRY *(Day 6)*

> 3 ounces lean flank steak, cut into thin 2-inch-long
>   strips
> ¼ cup sliced onion
> ¼ cup sliced bell pepper (optional)
> ¼ cup sliced mushroom
> ¼ cup shredded celery
> ¼ cup bean sprouts
> ¼ cup shredded carrots

¼ cup snow peas

SAUCE:
⅓ cup fat-free chicken broth
1 tablespoon dry sherry
1 tablespoon cornstarch
1 tablespoon light soy sauce
1 cup rice, steamed or boiled

Brown beef strips in skillet (or wok) coated with nonstick vegetable spray. When the beef is done, place it in a bowl. Add onion, bell pepper (optional), and mushroom to the skillet and sauté for 5 minutes, or until the onions are tender and translucent. Next add the chopped celery, bean sprouts, and carrots, cooking for another 3 to 4 minutes.

Combine sauce ingredients. Put meat back in skillet, stirring in snow peas and sauce. Cook for 5 minutes over medium heat, stirring frequently and making sure the sauce thickens somewhat. Serve on a bed of rice.

CHUCK ROAST *(Day 7)*

1 pound extra-lean beef chuck, fat trimmed
2 small onions, quartered
½ teaspoon salt
⅛ teaspoon pepper
1 cup fat-free beef broth (see Note)
6 new potatoes, halved
8 whole carrots, skinned
8 whole celery stalks

Season beef chuck with salt and pepper, and cook in beef broth in casserole pan for 2 to 2½ hours, or until tender. Add potatoes and vegetables after 1 hour, depending on desired firmness. One serving size is 4 ounces.

NOTE: *You can substitute for the fat-free broth, regular broth that's been heated, cooled, and fat skimmed off the surface.*

QUICK PIZZA *(Day 9)*

> 9 tablespoons store-bought pizza sauce
> 3 slices English muffin
> 3 slices nonfat cheese
> 1 1-ounce slice 98% fat-free presliced deli ham, chopped
> 1 ounce turkey salami, chopped
> Diced olives and bell pepper to taste

Spread 3 tablespoons sauce over each muffin slice, then top with cheese, meat, and vegetables. Toast until sauce is heated and cheese is fully melted.

BEEF STEW *(Day 10)*

> ½ pound bottom round steak, cut into cubes
> 1 cup sliced onion
> 1 cup carrot chips
> ½ cup chopped celery
> 4 new potatoes, quartered
> 2 cups fat-free beef broth (see Note)
> 4 tablespoons flour
> Salt and pepper to taste

Sauté beef chunks in skillet coated with nonstick vegetable spray over medium-low heat for about 30 minutes. Add onion and continue cooking for another 30 minutes, or until the meat is tender and browned, about 1 hour. Then add remaining vegetables and potatoes; simmer for 20 to 30 minute. Stir in 1½ cups broth. Stir flour into remaining ½ cup of broth, which you then pour into the stew. Let stew simmer for 5 to 10 minutes, or until broth thickens. Sprinkle salt and pepper to taste.

NOTE: *Instead of fat-free broth, you can use regular broth that's been cooled and had the fat skimmed off surface.*

CHICKEN FAJITAS *(Day 13)*

> *4 ounces skinless chicken-breast strips*
> *½ onion, sliced*
> *½ bell pepper, sliced*
> *2 12-inch wheat- or white-flour tortillas, warmed*

Chicken strips can be cooked by wrapping them in aluminum foil and banking them for 1 hour at 400° F. Sauté onion and bell pepper in a skillet coated with nonstick vegetable spray until they begin to brown. Then add chicken strips and continue to sauté until onions and peppers are done. Serve on heated tortillas.

BRAWNY BURRITO *(Day 14)*

See recipe for Day 12 lunch, adding one extra tortilla.

VEGETABLE BEEF SOUP *(Day 18)*

> *6 ounces lean top round steak*
> *6 ounces fat-free beef broth (see Note)*
> *1 potato, peeled, boiled, and diced*
> *1 cup chopped celery*
> *2 cups shredded carrot*
> *¾ cup chopped onion*
> *1 cup green beans, steamed*
> *1 cup chopped and stewed tomato*
> *Garlic powder and salt to taste*

Broil steak, then cut into small pieces and put into broth. Then add potato, celery, carrot, beans, and tomatoes. Simmer for 1 hour before mixing in the onion, garlic powder, and salt. *One serving is 3 cups.*

NOTE: *Instead of buying fat-free broth, you can use regular broth that's been cooled and had the fat skimmed off surface.*

SLOPPY JOE *(Day 20)*

> ½ *medium-size onion, diced*
> 1 *pound extra-lean ground round (no more than 15%*
>   *fat)*
> 2 *tablespoons chili sauce*
> ½ *cup ketchup or barbecue sauce*
> 1 *whole-grain bun, sliced*

Sauté diced onion in a skillet coated with nonstick vegetable spray, adding meat when the onion is tender. While meat begins to brown, stir in chili sauce and ketchup or barbecue sauce. Serve meat on bun.

QUESADILLAS *(Day 21)*

> 2 *slices nonfat cheese*
> 2 *12-inch wheat- or white-flour tortillas*
> *Diced onion and sliced jalapeño pepper to taste*
> ½ *cup Rosarita vegetarian refried beans, heated*

Arrange 1 slice of cheese on each tortilla, and roll them up (using toothpicks to hold them together, if necessary). Fry (nonstick vegetable spray only) until cheese melts and tortillas are fairly crisp. Serve with heated refried beans.

SOFT TACOS *(Day 22)*

> *Taco seasoning (in pouch)*
> 2 *ounces extra-lean ground round (no more than 15%*
>   *fat)*
> 2 *12-inch wheat- or white-flour tortillas, heated*
> 1 *ounce low-fat Cheddar, such as Lifetime, grated*
> *Diced tomato and onion*
> *Shredded lettuce*
> ½ *cup Rosarita vegetarian refried beans, heated*

Follow directions on taco seasoning pouch to cook beef. Add browned meat to heated tortillas, then top with Cheddar, tomato, onion, and lettuce. Serve with refried beans.

SWEDISH MEATBALLS (Day 23)

> 2 pounds extra-lean (no more than 15% fat) ground round
> 1 onion, diced
> 4 egg whites, or ½ cup Egg Beaters egg substitute
> 1 teaspoon salt
> ¼ teaspoon pepper
> 1 teaspoon paprika
> ½ cup 1% low-fat milk
> 1½ cups bread crumbs
> 1 cup mashed potatoes made with 1% low-fat milk and butter substitute
>
> SAUCE:
> ¼ cup water
> 1 10-ounce can consommé
> ¼ cup flour
> 1 cup nonfat sour cream

To make meatballs, mix beef, onion, egg whites, salt, pepper, paprika, milk, and bread crumbs in a large bowl. Then shape into 3-ounce meatballs and brown in a skillet coated with nonstick vegetable spray.

To make the sauce, mix together water and consommé, adding flour so it can dissolve. Stir over medium-low heat until thickened, then add sour cream. Stir until well mixed. Do not boil.

In another pan add meatballs and sauce, and bake at 325° F. for 1 hour. *One serving equals six 3-ounce meatballs.*

LEAN MEAT LOAF (Day 26)

> 2 pounds extra-lean (no more than 15% fat) beef
> 1½ cups rolled oats

1 ½ cups diced onion
4 egg whites, beaten together
1 teaspoon salt
⅛ teaspoon garlic powder

In a large bowl, mix all ingredients. Then put meat in a baking pan sprayed with nonstick vegetable spray, and bake for 60 to 90 minutes at 350° F. *One serving equals 2 half-inch slices of loaf.*

BEEF, CHEESE AND NOODLE CASSEROLE *(Day 27)*

8 ounces dry macaroni
8 ounces extra-lean (no more than 15% fat) ground beef
4 tablespoons flour
2 cups 1% low-fat milk
1 tablespoon Heartwise margarine
1 teaspoon salt
12 slices Kraft nonfat presliced cheese

Boil noodles until tender while browning beef in another pan sprayed with nonstick vegetable spray. Mix flour into milk along with Heartwise (not Heart Beat) margarine and salt. Stir over medium-low heat until thickened. Then add cheese slices and stir until cheese is melted and blended in.

Mix cooked macaroni and beef in a casserole dish (again, use nonstick vegetable spray), and pour cheese sauce over them. Bake in preheated oven at 350° F. for 15 to 20 minutes. *One serving size is 2 cups.*

BEEF STROGANOFF *(Day 29)*

1 ½ pounds lean (no more than 15% fat) ground beef
1 teaspoon salt
½ teaspoon ground black pepper

½ teaspoon garlic powder
½ teaspoon dried minced onion
2 tablespoons flour
1 11½-ounce can condensed cream of mushroom soup
1 2-ounce can mushrooms, including juice
1 cup nonfat sour cream
5 ounces fettucine noodles

Combine meat, salt, pepper, garlic powder, onion, and flour in skillet coated with nonstick vegetable spray, and cook until meat is fairly browned. Add undiluted condensed soup and simmer until all contents in the skillet become hot. Do not boil. Mix in mushrooms and sour cream just before serving. Cook the fettucine noodles, balancing your time so that you'll be done boiling the noodles by the time the beef is ready. Put Stroganoff over a bed of noodles on a plate. *One serving size is: ¼ recipe.*

CHAPTER EIGHT

Back on Track:
A Walking-Based Program
that You
Can Participate In

"Walking is man's best medicine"
—HIPPOCRATES

Some form of physical exercise *has* to play a part in your man's weight-loss program. Simply cutting back on the excess fat in his diet will take off his extra pounds, but the addition of some minimal physical exertion is far more effective than dietary changes alone for both his immediate and long-term goals of taking weight off and keeping it off.

Fortunately, most men will embrace the idea of exercising once they are reintroduced to it. Unfortunately, most of them will immediately do the wrong kind of exercise: they'll inevitably choose jogging or tennis or some other strenuous activity that bangs their bones around when the best physical medicine they can take is also the simplest: walking. And you can play a significant role in having your man realize just that.

Walking, believe it or not, is the best exercise with which to lose weight, and it has the same cardiovascular benefits as seemingly more strenuous activities. And that's true for women as well as men. But let's compare what goes on in your man's body with the most popular weight-loss activity, running/jogging, as opposed to walking, since I find that women have a hard time believing walking is the best of the fat-burning activities.

WEIGHT LOSS, WALKING AND RUNNING

When a man of any age or weight first heads out on a morning jog, he will quickly start burning calories—but calories of all types, not just those all-important calories from fat. If his average jogging time is forty-five minutes at a moderate pace, he will burn up all of his available blood sugar, then his body will use up its small supply of *glycogen*, an additional source of sugar/energy stored in the muscles. Only *after* the last of his glycogen is burned up will his body begin to think of burning fat as an additional source of fuel.

But that process doesn't commence easily. First his body has to convert the flab stored around his waist or chest into *free fatty acids*, which are then used as fuel to keep his run going. All this takes time—and in the interim he will struggle to keep up his pace, and be in something close to agony. Professional athletes and highly experienced runners have a variety of tricks to keep up their speed, including the practice of "carbo-loading," where they'll stuff themselves with high-carbohydrate foods in the days and weeks before a competition, in order to increase their store of glycogen and their physical endurance.

Your man probably won't take the idea of running competition that seriously. What he'll do is *stop*, since his body is telling him he can't run any farther, and he will feel he's done enough work. In a way he's right. But that doesn't change the fact that he has done very little to take off any of his excess pounds. His cardiovascular system (heart, lungs, and circulation) have benefited and the muscles in his legs and backside have gotten a nice workout—but he hasn't burned nearly the amount of fat he imagines he has. In fact, a forty-five-minute run at 4 miles per hour (a pretty average job) will burn only 300 calories of fat. At that rate, it would take a daily run for *two weeks* to burn a pound of fat. The same is true of swimming as it relates to fat burning.

Walking, however, is very different—and far more effective when it comes to losing weight. When he walks at a moderate pace on flat terrain—it shouldn't be that strange-looking "power walk" that a lot of people are doing nowadays and it shouldn't be up a steep hill—he sets pretty much every one of the hundreds of muscles and bones in his body into motion. His body will begin burning sugar for energy, as it does when he jogs, but for a variety of physiological reasons that probably go back to the days when we were hunter-gatherers and had to preserve our energy for long hauls through the woods, he will stop burning his blood sugar and switch to fat for fuel just ten minutes into his walk. When he's walking, a man doesn't have to go through the kind of complicated fuel-conversion process that running requires. When he's walking, he won't be aware of a thing; no exhaustion, no urge to call it quits. From the time he is reaching that key marker of ten minutes, he is sending the spare tire around his waist the same way wood in your fireplace goes—up in flames.

ADDED BENEFITS

Walking, unlike running, will also improve his posture, since he's probably gotten a little round-shouldered from years of sitting behind a desk, the wheel of a car, or in front of a television. Walking works the two major abdominal muscle groups as well, helping to tone the stomach muscles as the fat around his gut disappears. That can be an important factor in ridding him of a paunch, since other muscles, the hip flexors, have often taken over from the underused abdominals, causing his back to arch and his belly to stick out even more. Running does none of this.

WHY MEN WILL CHOOSE RUNNING—IF THEY'LL EXERCISE AT ALL

Despite the practical benefits I've just pointed out, you'll find that your man, if he opts for any exercise at all, will tend to choose running.

Why? The answer goes back to everything I talked about in Chapters 2 and 3. Since he still thinks of himself as a slender-waisted young guy, he will want to harken back to the days he spent running around the track as an eighteen-year-old, thinking that after ten or fifteen years spent in the front seat of the car and in the den lounger, he can just get out there and do it again. But he can't, and all your good work of getting him to eat differently will likely be for naught—because it's the rare man who can take weight off and keep it off without giving some sort of exercise a permanent place in his schedule.

There's also a sense of immediate gratification men get from running that they don't get from walking, until they realize what dramatic results walking can give. It's not the possibility of weight loss that concerns men—although they are convinced that running will help them achieve that. Running gives them a combination of pleasure and pain that appeals to their *macho* sensibilities. Pleasure from the famous endorphins (a natural pleasure-producing chemical manufactured by the brain during intense physical activity) is balanced by the pain from muscles that have been pressed into service too fast. It's that pain which convinces them that they're doing the right thing, when in fact a daily thirty- to forty-five-minute walk will take much more weight off them.

EXERCISE HE SHOULDN'T DO

You would be wise to discourage him from taking up running before he's lost a significant amount of weight and gotten in some walking experience. It isn't just that he won't lose weight as quickly as he will through walking; he also stands to hurt himself.

Vincent DeSouza

After I'd lost 10 of the 50 pounds I was trying to drop the first time around, I bought one of those expensive jogging suits, along with the $80 running shoes that I had to have to go with it. I started right away doing 3 miles, four times a week. At first it felt just great to be out there—it felt like college again—but that didn't last long. After about two weeks I couldn't take it anymore and I stopped. I was in so much pain in the morning that I had trouble moving my foot from the accelerator to the brake pedal without groaning. I guess twenty years of stuffing myself and never getting any exercise took its toll.

When the average overweight man past thirty (who's 30 to 50 pounds over a healthy weight) heads out on his first morning jog, eyes shining, endorphins starting to flow, he's hitting each of his soft, pudgy feet with *four times* his body weight, alternately, for every step of his run. That repetitive motion can do some real physical damage. Shin splints—microscopic tears in the tendons and muscle tissue surrounding the shin bone—often develop after a few weeks of this kind of punishment. If he ever had a knee injury, it will kick up again. If he never had one, he'll probably develop one. Arthritis can occur, due to all the pressure on his joints, as well as lower back pain.

Not to forget, too, that during the early stages of his weight loss, he's not going to be the most graceful thing in a pair of sneakers. The extra weight makes him unwieldy and the lack of recent experience with exercise will make him prone to accidents when he undertakes something that requires the coordination of running. Torn Achilles tendons, muscle pulls, and other musculoskeletal injuries are all common afflictions of the overweight man who takes up strenuous exercise instead of walking in order to lose weight.

He may grin and bear it, and even get a kick out of playing the injured sports hero for a while, but within a few weeks after starting his running routine, you will more than likely find the overpriced running shoes thrown in the closet, the jogging suit hanging from a nearby hook, and him parked back in front of the television set, dead set against any further physical exertion. So it's best to discourage this kind of extreme behavior from the start—and get him out there hoofing it slow but sure, preferably with you at his side making sure he doesn't goof off.

AN EXERCISE HE WON'T DO

If you're trying to think of some other alternative to running and other strenuous exercise in lieu of or in addition to walking, abandon the thought. Not only is walking by far the best weight-loss activity, bar none, in the world of physical fitness, it's also simple and you don't need special clothes (aside from a good pair of shoes and a jacket in winter) to do it.

The great mistake many active women make is thinking that they can get their man into an aerobics class with them. They're tempted by the thought that they can both go together, learn together—maybe even lose together. Unfortunately, that's almost never the case.

HARRY SHIVELY

My sister, Marie, got me to go to one of those aerobics classes when we both decided we should lose a few pounds. I don't know what I was thinking of. I got there and it was *all* women, in tights, jumping up, down, and sideways to music. That part of it was bad enough, but then I couldn't keep up with them. I was breathing hard ten minutes into an hour-long-session, and I never felt so uncoordinated in my life. Most of the others were nice, but the woman next to me finally said, "Would you mind keeping track of your backside?" after I'd rammed her with it a couple of times. I finally called it quits and slunk out of there after half an hour. My legs hurt for a week afterward.

Harry is one of the few men I've known who even ventured into an aerobics class, and the only reason he did it was because he didn't ask another man about it first. Your man most likely associates aerobics with a lot of women in leotards dancing and also with the possibility of making of fool of himself, the latter especially terrifying him more than anything else in the world, especially if he's overweight. Also, even a moderately difficult aerobics class is just too strenuous for him and can result in the same sort of injuries that come from running.

THE GYM MEMBERSHIP

Many women will also try an alternative route: buying their man a membership at a flashy health club and presenting it at Christmas or on his birthday.

Health club memberships are a fine idea—but again, only after he's taken some weight off and feels more confident about his physical self again. Health clubs, as many of you know, call pull the rug out from under the most self-confident overweight man.

HAL GREENBAUM

When I first made the decision to get rid of my gut, my wife Evelyn came home with a surprise: a health club membership for the two of us. I went twice, I think. It was too depressing seeing all those guys who were ten or fifteen years younger than me, looking better than I ever had. They all had stomachs like centipedes and I looked like a baby rhinoceros. And there were too many mirrors.

Men, as you know, have incredibly sensitive egos, and an experience like Hal's is enough to put many of them right back on the road to the refrigerator door. Give him six months of walking and eating right before you try the health club route. And who knows? But then he might be buying you a membership.

OTHER EXERCISE OPTIONS FOR HIM

Swimming, while a good muscle-toning and cardiovascular exercise, also doesn't have nearly the weight-loss power of walking. And, even if he denies he's overweight, you'll find that he's as enthusiastic about donning his swim trunks in front of strangers as he is about putting on a pair of spandex tights and going to an aerobics class.

Golf is a great walking exercise, but any suggestion from you about him taking it up should come after, not before, you get him on that three-to-five-times-a-week walking schedule. And no golf carts.

In general, things such as stationary bikes (outdoor cycling requires a measure of coordination that he won't have until he's shed some pounds), stairclimbers, and other at-home or gym means of getting in shape are fine. Lightweight lifting whether with free weights or with the guided weight machines that health clubs have (and that you can buy for at-home use) is very beneficial for improving appearance and developing strength *after* he's made some progress downsizing. But to maximize results and minimize the twin risks that he'll resume his old lifestyle or hurt himself trying to do too much too soon, you have to start him out walking.

Sex is actually a pretty good fat burner, too, if you get enough of it. Somebody did a study a few years back and figured out that you burn about 300 calories an hour during an "average" lovemaking session, which isn't bad, if you can manage it once a day. And one of the few benefits of the aging libido is that it will take him longer, so he'll burn more fat calories.

AT THE STARTING LINE

Almost at the same time you begin talking to him about food and his eating habits, as well as the special male physical problems you've read about here, gently bring up the facts about men and walking that you now know. Also, give some thought to small ways in which you can begin to get him upright, out of his chair and *ambulatory*.

EVELYN GREENBAUM

I found that with the new low-fat breakfast I was making in the morning, Hal and I actually had a little bit more time together than we did when I was cooking a big breakfast. I made sure I needed something from the store at the corner at least three mornings a week and I told Hal I didn't want to walk down there alone—it was about a quarter of a mile each way. And I'd always insist on walking. He huffed and puffed at first, but he gradually got used to it and we started making a circle around the neighborhood at night, too, with the dog. That was three years and 35 pounds ago for him, and now I can't keep him still. He's always out playing handball or tennis or something else. I think the walking got him accustomed to using his body again, and he was happy to find it still worked pretty well.

The small things *do* add up when it comes to exercise. Do anything that comes to your mind to get him in motion. When you go out together, urge him to park some distance away from your destination so you'll both have to walk to get there. Insist on taking the stairs instead of elevators and escalators—just anything that involves putting one foot in front of the other. It all counts.

THE EVENING WALK

One of the most beneficial walking activities you can initiate is to simply ask him to walk with you in the evening, right after dinner. Most men will be far more willing to engage in any physical activity at that time of day, and fat-burning benefits aside, a good long walk is a wonderful way to shake off the stresses of the day. It's also essential that you accompany him, because men will use the boredom that accompanies solitary walking to call it quits early—or slip into the donut shop at the corner for some well-deserved (in his mind) fat fuel. Most couples grow closer together as a result of these walks, because it's an ideal time to discuss your relationship, job worries, children, noisy neighbors—all the things that you never seem to be able to make room for.

LINDA REARDON

Joe was a Type-A lawyer and he had already had one heart attack. The walking wasn't my idea, it was his doctor's, and there really wasn't much choice about him doing it—forty-five minutes, every weekday night, moderate pace, was the order.

I went with him, to make sure he actually walked. At first he kind of stomped through it—like most lawyers, he's not fond of being told what to do. But after a week or two, we both began to look forward to it. It gave us an opportunity to talk, which we hadn't really done in years. It was practical, too. We decided things about the kids, where we were going financially, a lot of things. Even today, although Joe's in good physical shape, we're still out there, rain or shine.

You don't have to walk in the pouring rain, like Linda and Joe, but you shouldn't let winter stop you, either. There's nothing wrong with a little cold, as long as you're bundled up properly. But failing that, get in the car and drive down to the local mall and walk up, down, and around until you think you've gotten in forty-five minutes worth. To add some variety and meet your three-to-five-times-a-week walking mandate, scout out shopping areas other than your usual one and plan to substitute indoor places such as museums, auto shows—anything that will keep him on his feet—for the weekends.

An added medical benefit to the afterdinner walk that few people know and fewer people discuss: walking aids the digestive system. By gently massaging his whole food-processing factory, walking offers a perfectly natural afterdinner antacid, provided his water and fiber intake are adequate.

THE WALKING FACTS

The average overweight man should walk at least a mile, three to five times a week. That schedule will aid his low-fat eating program considerably, and can mean the difference between his losing 1 or 2 pounds per week. But he must keep up a minimum of thirty minutes of foot to pavement, which will let him cover a mile. Within two weeks of initiating your walking schedule with him, though, you should try to work up to forty-five minutes.

Pace. There are many speeds at which you can walk. Most fitness professionals define them as:

- *casual strolling*—a very relaxed pace, like what you'd do window shopping. Too slow for cardiovascular benefits for him, but fast enough to burn a considerable amount of fat, if he keeps going for the recommended time length.
- *functional walking*—the pace you'd use walking from one place to another, about twice the speed of strolling, 2 to 4 miles per hour.
- *brisk walking*—just what it says, and has considerable fat-burning capability at a speed of 3.5 to 5.5 miles per hour.

- *race walking*—almost competitive, often done at more than 5.5 miles per hour. It's almost impossible to maintain a normal conversation while race walking.
- *weight-loaded walking*—a race walk done while the walker is loaded down with weights. Walking with weights can throw your muscles and joints out of whack, and it's certainly not for your man if he hasn't exercised in a long time.

You'll want to start out having him walk at a casual stroll, and work up to at least a functional walk within a couple of weeks. If you both feel like walking briskly after a while, fine, but I've learned that with men and walking, just to have them out there doing it in those first few months is enough. As long as he's out there walking three times a week for at least a half hour, he's going to reap fitness and weight-loss benefits whether he's moving fast or slow.

FINE POINTS OF WALKING

Some walking specialists emphasize taking your own pulse at several points during the walk; achieving target heart rates; and stretching before, after, and during the walk. That's all very nice, but he's just not going to do it, unless he's already a convinced health and fitness fan—in which case you wouldn't need this book. In my view, the only time any of these things is necessary is if he has serious health problems (such as heart disease or extreme obesity—more than 100 pounds above his ideal body weight) that exercise can affect, in which case he should be closely monitored. But those are rare cases. I think that if you can get him out there and moving, and understand how far you can go and when, you'll be accomplishing a worthwhile goal and you shouldn't worry about somewhat fussy details. I'll guarantee you, at some point after the first three months, he'll pick up the pace himself.

Sam Hall

I was going on sixty when my daughter finally got me to go walking with her every afternoon about 3:00. We'd go down to the high school playing field and back—about a mile and a half,

158 HOW TO HELP YOUR MAN LOSE WEIGHT

altogether. I did lose some of the weight the doctor told me to get rid of, but something else happened, too. I got such a kick from the realization that my body still *worked* that I started taking up other things as well. I picked up a tennis racket for the first time in thirty years, and now I can beat my son-in-law, most of the time, anyway. I joined the municipal golf club, too.

OTHER PRACTICAL FACTS

Good walking shoes are the one piece of special equipment you should consider buying him. Walking in business shoes that are too tight and stiff, or leisure shoes that just don't provide enough support (and leave the foot too close to the pavement), will put a crimp into his walking/weight–loss campaign very quickly; blisters, aching feet, and other aches and pains can develop with incredible speed if he's not wearing a proper walking shoe. Altogether there are a number of shoes on the market designed specifically for walking (and they are superior to nonwalking shoes), you should generally look for shoes with:

- a leather upper (provides a good fit for the bone structure of your foot)
- a firm heel support (the back of the shoe—to prevent blisters and chafed skin)
- a slightly elevated heel
- flexibility where the ball of the foot meets the toes (his foot should be able to bend)
- a squarish front, so his toes have some breathing space and aren't repeatedly jammed against the front of the shoe while he's walking
- a relatively thick—but still flexible—sole to protect against the pebbles, rocks, and sticks that you'll both be stepping on
- laces that pull up snugly without being too tight.

He'll also need some thick socks to protect further the sole of the foot from injury. You don't want him to have the smallest physical reason for quitting your walking routine.

HIPPOCRATES WAS RIGHT

The facts and myths about walking that I've described are intended to provide you with the knowledge to get him started on a walking program. If he embraces the new eating and living style that this book is intended to bring both of you, he'll add other activities within a few months, he'll learn (or relearn, in many cases) the benefits of healthier eating and exercise—without becoming a vegetarian or a triathlete. Research shows that adult men who stick to some form of substantial physical exercise for more than six months after emerging from slothfulness are likely to keep it up for the rest of their lives. That's good news for both of you.

PART THREE

LIFE WITH
THE THIN MAN

CHAPTER NINE

Keeping Him Trim: Weight-Maintenance Tips For the Long Haul

It's an unfortunate fact, but a fact nonetheless, that 90 percent of men who lose gain back their lost weight within twenty-four months. And of those 90 percent, most will gain back some additional weight as well.

Your man may regain his unwanted weight for a variety of reasons. He may not have completely changed his thinking about his relationship with eating and exercise, and slide back to the old habits without realizing that damage done once can be done twice. He may fall victim to the winter holidays—traditionally the most dangerous time of year for the newly thin, with a danger zone that extends from October through the New Year. Well-meaning and not so well-meaning saboteurs may lead him astray.

What can you do without watching him every minute? Plenty. But you've got to start while you're helping him lose the first time around.

BEGIN AT THE BEGINNING

Your educational role during your man's weight loss is extremely important for long-term maintenance as well as for your 163 initial campaign to slim him down. Why? Because one of the most important reasons for the high failure rate among men on traditional diet programs is their perspective on the weight-loss *process*. As I have said in previous chapters, men tend to be project-oriented in general—that is, they believe that all life's endeavors have a beginning, a middle, and an end, much like mowing the lawn, changing the spark plugs, making a business deal, or trying and adjudicating a legal case.

SID WEINTRAUB

When I started on a liquid diet for the first time, I thought, "Oh, it's only for six weeks and then I can go back to *normal*." Normal meant blinis with butter and cheese, corned beef for lunch—the whole high-fat trip. So I suffered through those six weeks, breathed a sigh of relief, and then I felt entitled to go back to my favorite foods. And it only took me another *eight* weeks to put back on all the weight I'd lost in six.

What you have to do to keep him on the straight and narrow is initiate a variety of changes in your life together that will help ensure his fitness on a permanent basis—but do it early on in your campaign to help him lose. You should never stop talking to him about the permanence of the changes he's making. Don't harp, but bring the subject up every couple of days for at least six months. Don't buy packaged foods or drink that will lead him to believe that "it'll all be over" in a few weeks. I have found that the men who stay with a changed diet and who keep some kind of regular exercise in their lives for six months are more likely to make those changes a permanent feature of their lifestyle landscape.

The 30-Day Meal Plan outlined in Chapter 7 makes your task a little easier, because when following it he will have no reason to feel deprived of any of his favorite foods. And if he slides back on one or two food items once in a great while, that's no sin: too much eating inflexibility has been the shoals of many a weight-maintenance program.

FLEXIBILITY IN FOOD

Don't be afraid of doing something different now and then, because everyone gets sick of the same old routine, whether it's high fat or low fat, or the disguised low-fat food that is the calling card of Chapter 7. I recommend that you go out and eat different types of food at least twice a month. Italian food (which is traditionally low-fat, if you have the pasta without the meatballs and avoid Americanized Italian food that's loaded down with high-fat cheese), Chinese, and Mexican are favorites of mine, and they'll satisfy his yen for something different without rekindling a desire for fat and sugar. But you can really try almost any type of cuisine, outside of high-fat Northern European fare, once both of you gain a basic sense of what is high-fat and what isn't, and once he is weaned off of a regular high-fat diet with an eating program that doesn't starve him. One of the reasons men gain back weight so quickly is that most "diets" deprive them of carbohydrates, so they go on a binge after the diet is "over."

VARIETY IN EXERCISE

The six-month mark with his walking/exercise regimen is especially important. Research has proven that men who stay with a regular program of exercise are far more likely to keep fit for the rest of their lives than men who exercise intermittently, a fact which will enable you to stay home without worrying that he's going to walk as far as the nearest bakery. At that twenty-four-week point, it seems that men become accustomed to the renewed sense of energy and well-being that go with the flow of endorphins we were talking about in Chapter 8, and you may have more trouble keeping him off his feet than on them. Boredom can still be a problem, however.

JOSEPH SMITH

You can only walk around the same high school track so many times, and frankly I got a little antsy hoofing it around the same circle over and over again. That's when my wife suggested that we start getting involved in some other things. She bought me a tennis racket the Christmas after I knocked off 30 pounds, and we both took lessons and started playing twice a week.

I discussed the importance of a varied walking routine in Chapter 8, and variety assumes greater importance in the months following his slim-down. He will have to refill the time he previously spent eating, and you can help him find healthful activities to do that.

He doesn't necessarily have to pound the pavement, hit a ball, pump a stack of iron, or otherwise burn calories in order to contribute to his weight-loss maintenance. There are plenty of other activities that will keep his mind off food. New hobbies play an extremely important part here. Think of one that would interest him and encourage him in it. It could be anything from stamp collecting to collecting classic cars—as long as it doesn't take place near a refrigerator and involves more effort than pressing the remote button for the television. It sounds corny, but parlor games are a great way to keep occupied. Chess, checkers, and cards keep his hands too busy to lift food from snack tray to mouth.

If he doesn't backslide, as mentioned before, your man will be naturally inclined to take on more and more physical activities—especially as he becomes more self-confident about his appearance and his physical abilities. You can encourage him by buying him a health club membership or home gym equipment—that you can use too—and encouraging participation in weekend sports from elitist sailing to working man's bowling.

THE AGING MALE BODY

Don't be concerned about him becoming more physically vulnerable as he ages. A man's metabolic rate doesn't really change significantly until he reaches his late sixties, so he can keep up tennis, golf, or a variety of fairly strenuous activities, just about as well at sixty as he did at thirty-five. And he should do just that.

FREDERICK WHITLOW

The stress of my law practice had turned me into a 275-pound compulsive eater and chain smoker by the time I was forty years old. Caroline, my wife, persuaded me to lose and begin an exercise program by telling me she wanted me to go down to the local funeral home—some friends of ours own it—and pick out my own coffin. I lost over 75 pounds and took up racquetball three times a week. I still play a pretty good game, twenty-five years later.

Your man's dietary needs will remain fairly constant, barring any specific medical problems, and he doesn't have to change the number of calories he's taking in as he ages, as long as he's not gaining any weight. He should, however, always remember that magical number, 30 *percent calories from fat* and never go beyond it. And if he does gain weight, I wouldn't blame the aging process as the likeliest culprit. I would take a close look to see if he's falling off the healthy weight wagon in some other way, like cheating. If he does cheat, and you suspect it, address the issue directly. Everybody makes a mistake, you can tell him, but the sooner you correct it, the easier the mistake is rectified.

THE SEDUCTIVE HOLIDAY SEASON

If you keep a little variety in his (and your) eating and exercise life, his weight maintenance will not present an overpowering dilemma, long-term. However, it's not just you and him against the world. There are other factors that affect his ability to keep weight off; time of year and relatives, co-workers and friends are first among them.

CHRISTMAS BEGINS IN SEPTEMBER

Although holidays like Memorial Day, the Fourth of July, and Labor Day will present him with considerable temptation to go back to high-fat foods, they're still just a few days and usually just a few bad meals: a hot dog or a full-bodied beer won't kill him, or blow him back up to his old weight. But even with this single episode, don't be afraid to mention it to him and point out the harm that he will do to himself if he keeps it up.

It's not long after Labor Day, however, that the most dangerous temptation for an overweight man makes its yearly appearance: Halloween selling season. It's when those big bags of little candy bars that are supposed to go to the neighborhood kids for Halloween appear, until the last lyric of "Auld Lang Syne" fades into the cold New Year's Day air, that his weight willpower is most severely tested.

HALLOWEEN ISN'T ONLY FOR KIDS

Selling Halloween candy six weeks before the hobgoblins actually arrive is not something supermarkets do for your convenience. Candy companies seem to know that most of that Halloween candy they send to the store will never see the inside of a witch's or mini-ghost's bag: The man in your house will doubtless eat it all well before they ever get a crack at it. Then, as the marketeers expect, you'll have to go out and buy more. The businessmen have successfully convinced you that you need to buy the candy early in order to be "prepared." Many times, you'll put the candy in a dish near the door weeks before the kids are supposed to arrive. Again, they'll never see it. And then you buy more—and more. Of course, the holiday comes and goes, there probably weren't as many kids as you expected, so the man of the house takes it upon himself to finish the leftovers.

A PLUNGE INTO THE TRADITIONAL GRAVY BOAT

With Halloween over, his battle against bad eating weakens. By early November he will adopt a what-the-hell attitude about eating and drinking over the upcoming eight weeks, since he figures he can't win. And due to the food-oriented nature of Thanksgiving, Hanukkah, and Christmas, and the calorie/sugar–soaked alcohol glow that surrounds New Year's, he's *almost* right.

BEN PRIOLA

I'd been pretty good all year, since my wife and I decided that it wasn't in our interest to have me dead of a heart attack before I'd made my first million. I'd dropped 25 pounds. But when the two weeks before Thanksgiving rolled around, I was a goner. One party after another, a lot of extra food coming into the house—all of it for "company," of course. I didn't sit down and eat big meals like I'd done before. It was more of a slow and steady slide—some hot dogs wrapped in dough here, some Christmas cookies there. But, boy, did it add up. By New Year's Day, I'd gained back 15 of the 25 pounds I'd lost, and I found the prospect of going through all that dieting again pretty depressing, mostly because I was disappointed in my lack of willpower.

UN-HAPPY HOLIDAYS

Why does he weaken at this time of year? The endless round of parties, both at the workplace and at home, enforced social or family get-togethers, along with the financial pressures of gift-giving can make the "winter" holidays a stressful time for many men, and they cope with their anxiety by reaching for all too readily available snacks. These are also very much food holidays, as mentioned; that can be a fatal combination in a society that reaches for food in response to both stress *and* depression. But don't forget that we're *not* talking about one day here: it's actually a *three-month* stretch of overeating, from October 1 until January 1. That's 25 percent of his year spent overeating. And the toll on your man? The average male over thirty can easily gain between 15 and 20 pounds by January 2.

WHAT TO DO: JOYOUS BUT FAT-FREE HOLIDAY PLANNING

No one wants to be a food Scrooge when the holidays come around, and it's almost impossible to avoid some indulgence on his part. But, again, ignorance plays an important part in his year-end weight gain, so your educational abilities will once more come into play, along with some practical steps.

First, stop your habit of bringing Halloween candy into the house early, and consider giving away something else besides sugary treats to the neighborhood kids. As you know from chapter 6, sugar highs and lows are a surefire way to keep him overweight (or make him that way again), and you'll be doing the neighborhood mothers a favor as well. Give away fruit, sugarless gum—almost anything but those little fat-and-sugar missiles that come one hundred to the bag. And under any circumstances, don't put any snacks out in plain sight until October 30, at the earliest.

Around Halloween time, you should begin talking with him about the food risks associated with the holidays, and what they will present to the both of you as a challenge to resist temptation. A woman with a man who needs to drop some dangerous poundage usually doesn't want to be perceived as a nag, especially at a "happy" time of year. But there's a significant difference between nagging and helping—the latter practice never ends in an argument.

In order to minimize the temptations around him, you might think about maintaining as fat-proof a house as possible—come January 2, you'll be glad you did, for both your sakes. Substitute some of the snacks listed in Chapter 7 for the traditional high-fat treats, cut out the fat from gravies and other rich foods, and don't be afraid to carry your low-fat lifestyle to the holiday table, in the form of butter substitutes; skinless turkey; and sugar-free pies, cakes, and cookies. As for liquor, keep the supply as much out of sight as possible—don't put the bottles out in plain view, because that's an invitation to indulge.

I've said before that helping your man lose weight is an educational task, and it's not a part-time one, for him or for you. You both should agree well before the holidays on what kind of eating and drinking behavior will result in a truly happy New Year's Day, and what kind will result (for him) in anger, remorse, and a curse at his own puffy reflection in the mirror on the first day of a freshly minted year.

MARGE WAPNER

My brother, Fred, had been living with me for eight months—since he'd gotten divorced—and with the low-fat diet I had him on, plus a little bit of exercise every day, he'd gotten back the body he'd had ten years ago. But the holidays just ruined it all. I think it was a variety of reasons that made him do it; he was sad over not being with his family, everybody *else* was eating and drinking, so he gave in. And because it was cold, he had a good excuse for not taking his daily walk downtown and back after work.

By January 1 he was back up to his old weight, 210. And to top it all off, he woke up New Year's morning with a hangover, looking bloated and swearing he'd never do it again, of course. Some New Year's resolution.

EAT ALREADY! THE BENEVOLENT SABOTEURS

As we've been discussing, the holidays are one of the most dangerous times of year for the man trying to keep the weight off, and for you in your attempt to help him. In addition to the endless plates of food and bottles of liquor around the both of you, it's also the most active time of year for the friend or family member who'd rather have the fat man they knew before back in their life. And such well-meaning people are not at all reluctant to try to run roughshod over you to accomplish that goal.

It often comes in the form of his "favorite" dish suddenly making an appearance—whether you're visiting them or their visiting you. It could also be a warning to him about his health—usually given in a whisper when you're out of earshot ("You're looking a little thin"). Or maybe it's something a little more direct, like a hint that you're trying to get your hands on his life insurance (and the car payment book) by starving him to death.

DARLENE PESANELLI

Sam had lost about 40 pounds when his mother came on her annual holiday visit from back East. She'd barely gotten off the plane before she was telling him that it was nice he'd lost the weight and all that but he didn't look good. Then a big laugh and she's leaning over the front seat to hit me and ask why I was starving him to death. The next thing I knew, she was baking pies and cooking that fatty sausage she'd fed him when he was a kid. And he ate it all, of course—Joe always turned back into a ten-year-old around her. He gained back 10 pounds in the two weeks she was here.

FAMILY

Unfortunately, we can't choose our relatives, or in Darlene's case, our in-laws. They can be the worst weight saboteurs to confront your man, since they have an almost primal fear of seeing change in him. Why? In the case of close relatives, they often see your success in helping him slim down as a smack in the face, a kind of "*You* just didn't know how to treat him, but I do," statement. Then the inevitable rationalizations follow as the saboteur tells your man that he doesn't look good, that he's making himself sick—in short, all of the tricks that men have tried on dieting women for years, because *they* fear change!

Don't underestimate the power of saboteurs to undermine his otherwise successful maintenance program. Especially where family are concerned, there are many psychological factors, particularly guilt and a desire to please, that come into play, most often when you're not around.

DARYL MACAULAY

When I'd gone over to my dad's house after I'd finally gotten myself back into a size 34 pair of jeans, he'd always have my mother set out a big meal—just like when I was a kid. He'd never had much of a weight problem himself, like I did, and he never seemed to notice that my size had gotten out of hand. He wanted me to sit down and clean my plate like I'd always done, and imitate the way he ate. Since I always felt like a kid again when I was in their house, I did just that. Luckily they lived about an hour away, so it didn't do me any real harm because I didn't visit that often.

Daryl's wrong—going back to the same portions and fatty foods can whet his taste for more of the same; he's just lucky that his parents live at a safe distance. But suppose they move across the street?

A man can't rely on distance and other artificial solutions for an answer when what helps most with long-term weight maintenance is facing down any kind of temptation and making all other considerations—including parents—secondary to his health and well-being.

An open discussion of the damage these well-meaning saboteurs can cause is where you should start: tell him honestly what you've observed, how you think his weight and health are affected by his giving in to these folks on food issues. Ask him to consistently choose his own health over their "feelings," and then help him do it by backing him up in conversation or accompanying him when he goes to see them—and speaking up when you see dietary transgressions about to take place. At least for those critical first six months after he loses weight, play policewoman when you suspect saboteurs are prowling around, so his new eating style and exercise regimen have a chance to take firm hold.

DANA MACAULAY

I finally sat Daryl down and we talked about his family's food habits. His going over there and eating the same old fried foods was getting to be a problem, and I could see the weight creeping back slowly but surely. He mentioned his parents, but his two brothers lived right here in town, and they were always trying to stuff him as well as themselves.

During our talk, I said, "Here is the situation as I see it. . . ." and told him—without dragging his family through the mud—how I thought they were pushing him back toward the 200-pound mark. It was a good conversation for us, and he agreed. We made a pact as to how he would just stay with his new eating patterns when he was around them. But I made a point of going with him as often as possible when he headed over to their place. Then I hit on the idea of having them over here, so the food and drink would be under *our* control.

THE BEST BUDDY

Aside from his immediate family, your man's male friends present the most formidable obstacle to his permanent healthy eating habits. Traditions like the three-martini lunch, a ball game complete with hot dogs and beers, or a Saturday-morning visit to the donut shop are forms of male bonding that die hard. All you can do is present him with an informed choice to make—that he can't eat right 50 percent or even 75 percent of the time and expect to achieve long-lasting positive results.

I don't mean that you should try to stop outings with friends (and your company won't be as welcome as it is around his family), because then he'll starting associating his healthy body with the loss of his friends, and begin viewing thinness as punishment. But do suggest that he adjust important details of his outings. Example: He can go to a tavern after work or to a fine restaurant for lunch, but pass on the alcohol and high-fat foods. You can help him by researching and recommending a restaurant with at least some healthy choices on the menu. Emphasize that he has to stick to his guns, that it's a matter of his health. What I've found is that his true friends will eventually adjust to his new way of life and stop pressuring him—or just tease him in a good-natured way. Happily, some of his male friends will start feeling competitive about his fit form, too, and when they fail to knock him back to square one, they'll join him.

RAY TUCKEY

Howie and I used to have a standing date down at a local sports bar to watch Monday night football. There was a lot of beer, a lot of chips, all the things Ginny and I agreed wouldn't be a part of my life anymore. What I did was put the bowl of pretzels in front of me and ignore the chips, and switch from beer to Diet Coke. Howie thought it was a little strange at first—he hates any kind of change, but he stopped bugging me about it after a month or so. I think he was afraid I'd dump him along with my bad eating habits, and when that didn't happen, he was fine. Then I guess he started feeling a little bit self-conscious himself, because he started eating the same way I did, asking questions about how I'd lost weight. So he started coming with Ginny and me three times a week on our walks around the school track, and *he* got rid of his spare tire.

What Ray did was make *decisions* about his priorities in life. He decided that his focus was on the football game and the company of his friend, not the food and the booze, and Ginny helped him clarify the difference.

MAINTENANCE AND EVOLUTION

I've said an awful lot about *you* and about *him* as individuals, and how you affect each other. But aside from the practical considerations of the post-weight-loss period that we've just reviewed, there will be considerable change in another important area—the most important area—that you share: your *relationship*. Like your bodies and minds, it, too, will evolve as a result of your helping him to get healthy, in mostly welcome but even some unwelcome ways.

CHAPTER TEN

How Your Relationship Will Change as a Result of His Weight Loss

Presuming that your man listens to what you have to say about his weight, he'll have taken off a significant amount of poundage within four to six months of your working with him. That's when a new phase will begin for you: coping with your newly thin man and readjusting that thing that the two of you share: your *relationship*. You'll be more happy with some of the lifestyle and relationship changes that his new svelte shape will bring, but there are some potential pitfalls to dealing with the newly thin man that you should be aware of.

THE WOLF PHASE

After your man has reached a healthy weight, he will likely go through a phase (it usually lasts from sixty to ninety days) where he's a little *over*pleased with his physique—and with his newfound appeal to the opposite sex. Often, the workplace is where he stretches his newfound wolf's legs.

LINDA EVERS

> After Henry lost all his extra weight—he looked terrific, I have to say, even though he was over forty—he would come home from the office and say, "Well, Janie came by my office today and said *this* and Bonnie said *that* and she's so cute. . . ." It suddenly occurred to me that he'd worked at the same place eight years and this was the first time he'd *ever* mentioned any of these women; they wouldn't give him the time of day when his belly was hanging over his belt and now they couldn't get enough of him. It made me see red.

Linda's reaction is completely understandable, but in reality there's no need for her to be hostile. Because men, as they get older, don't usually associate the declining interest of women in them with their weight but rather their age (or sometimes their hairline), they're often more surprised and delighted with their newfound attractiveness than you might think. To them, it's truly a rebirth, much like stepping out into the spring air after a long winter's hibernation. They discover that they can still be flirtatious and get a response, or have someone do the same with them. But while I have seen many cases of a flirtatious man driving the permanent woman in his life crazy, I have rarely seen a case where a healthy relationship was torn apart by a man actually cheating on his wife after he loses weight. He'll get and give more attention to other women, but that's to be expected. If he's more attractive, he's going to attract more attention, and human beings being what they are, he's going to take some pleasure in basking in it, especially at first. After three months, at most, you'll observe that flirting will have lost its novelty value for him, and that you will be less sensitive when he gets a little too enthusiastic about what other women do or say about him. My advice? Wait him out on this one, and be glad that you have someone attractive again.

Strangely enough, I've seen many more relationships break up after the *woman* has lost weight rather than the man. I think this has more to do with the fact that the man (overweight or normal weight) usually hasn't been a part of the woman's weight-loss process. It's as though she is suddenly a different person, someone he doesn't know—and he'd rather have the overweight partner with whom he was secure. When she refuses to return to a way of life she hated, he jumps ship.

ON THE SEX FRONT

Overweight men, regardless of how many pounds above their ideal weight, usually make mediocre lovers, at best. That's not only because they (and probably you) are psychologically hamstrung by their weight, but because excess pounds affect so many of the body systems that control sexual performance. The function of the endocrine system is impaired, causing problems with male hormone production and resultant loss of libido, or sexual desire. Vascular, or blood flow, problems often result from his overweight, and can interfere with his ability to get and maintain an erection. Overweight and the sugar/alcohol problems I talked about in Chapter 6 also result in his being plain old worn out at day's end, like a work horse that's been pulling too heavy a load.

After he's back down to a normal weight, his libido will almost immediately spring back to life, so be ready for a rejuvenated mate in bed. Sex will be more frequent, more satisfying, and frankly, more aesthetically pleasing for you—very few women enjoy looking at a man with a big, bulbous paunch with his shirt *on*, never mind off. But an increased sexual appetite doesn't mean he's going to turn into a sexual compulsive, bothering you every minute; it simply means that you can resume a good, regular sex life with a partner who's in optimal health.

DEBBIE SUTTON

Jim and I had been together for nine years and to be honest, I'd forgotten what it was like to have a good time in bed. Jim was always too tired, asleep already, grouchy, groggy from stuffing himself, or something else. To make a long story short, we were down to once a month, and even that seemed like a chore.

When Jim got his high blood pressure diagnosis and lost 50

pounds, then it was another story. He'd come home from his nightly walk full of the right kind of energy and ready to go. When we got in the bedroom, it was like someone had turned the clock back to our first week together. I always assumed that our sex life was on a natural decline because we'd been together so long. But believe me, it doesn't have to be that way at all. I'm a firm believer now in good health *and* good sex.

THE CASTRATION COMPLEX

Sometimes, however, your man may have a difficult time, adjusting his sense of masculinity to the new reflection in the mirror. He still may be clinging to the concept of "big" as more manly, discussed in Chapter 3. He may be impaired sexually by a little performance anxiety, but you should be aware that this is most likely a psychological readjustment to his new size. Symptoms? Let one of my patients tell you.

Harriet Reed

Dan had lost about 55 pounds over the course of a year, which improved his blood pressure, but it sure didn't do much for his attitude. He would constantly complain that I'd bought him the wrong size clothes, and then he'd start in on how people around him weren't treating him with as much "respect" as they used to. I could see that he felt uncomfortable, despite all the positive changes I'd helped him make. In fact, he acted similar to the way a lot of women are made to feel when they're the least bit overweight. Needless to say, our sex life during that period was practically nonexistent.

Harriet, of course, couldn't imagine what was going through Dan's mind: all the fears of loss of masculinity because of his weight loss, years of training to assume that big is better. That deeply ingrained belief can affect his sexual performance and appetite, though, again, it's usually for a fairly short period of time: one to three months.

My advice to a woman who runs into these problems with her man is fairly simple: stick with him, and let him know on a regular basis—daily, if possible—for those first few months that *you* think he looks terrific. Make specific comments on his physique, how good he looks in his new clothes, and also connect the two—tell him those clothes he's just gotten set off his new body to advantage. He'll make his own connection before too long.

As far as the medical aspects of sex are concerned, if he has problems getting or keeping an erection on a regular basis, he should see a doctor about possible vascular problems. But if you think he's just a little uncertain of "the new him," be patient, encouraging—and maybe a little more aggressive in bed than in the past. Most men love it, and it will reinforce their sense of their own attractiveness.

YOUR MAN AS OVEREXERCISER

You might also find, after several months, that your man becomes something close to obsessive about exercising. Most often, the offending sport is running (although it can be almost anything else, weight lifting included), and the story among women with a newly active man is fairly similar.

SHARON KOSLOSKI

Jerry's weight came off pretty fast, and then he had such a morbid fear that he'd go back to being paunchy he took to the track morning and night. Then he started competing and I didn't even see him on the weekends. I got a little concerned because he started coming home with leg injuries. I started to think I was better off when he was heavier; at least then I had some company, even though I knew that was wrong. I didn't know what to do.

You have to remember that a man who's just gotten his body back into shape is undergoing some chemical reactions due to exercise (production of endorphins, mostly) that are a little bit addictive—he's really feeling *good*, physically, for the first time in a long while. Add to that the fact that he may also be undergoing something of a midlife crisis, and he now connects physical exercise to beating back the flab and paunch ravages of Father Time. He figures the more he does it, the younger he'll look. In dealing with him on this issue, you should ask yourself several questions:

- How severe is the problem? Does he completely ignore you in favor of his running? Or is he simply not around as much as you would like?
- Do you participate in his activities with him?
- Do you tend to treat him in the same way you did *before* he lost the weight?
- What are your own attitudes toward his weight loss?

In assessing the severity of the problem, you have to look closely at his behavior. In the rare cases I've seen where men will actually run on shin splints (inflamed tissue around the shin bone that's extremely painful) there were real psychological problems involved, and I recommend therapy. That kind of overexercising is obsessive/compulsive and should be brought to the attention of a professional.

As for the rest of my questions, if you find yourself answering any one of them with a "yes," you have to do again what I've advocated time and time again throughout this book: talk to him about it, and take an active stance in his physical life yourself. Tell yourself that you were a major force in bringing him this far, and that you shouldn't abandon him now. And think about joining him! It's another opportunity to be together, and everyone, including you, could use a little more exercise than they're getting.

TOM WATSON

I started running on a regular basis after I'd dropped my first 25 pounds. It felt terrific! Here I was at forty-three, after being told that there was a good chance that I'd drop dead from a heart attack before I'd turned fifty—and suddenly I was actually feeling more energetic after I'd been jogging around the track for a half hour. Not only that, but after I started competing in 10K races, I was competing against guys twenty years my junior. I even won once in a while, but frankly, that wasn't why I was doing it.

But my wife, Susan, got really ticked off that I was spending all this time at the track or away at races that I used to spend eating and drinking with her. She wasn't shy about telling me that, either, which was great. So I went out and got her six pairs of running shoes for her birthday, and we started running *together*.

Before you get too annoyed with him, think of what it feels like for a man who had ample evidence that he was past his prime forever, and then suddenly he feels good about his body again. It was only the extra weight that was making him feel old! Giving him that renewed sense of himself, after all, was part of your goal in helping him take it off. Remember, too, what kind of attitude he had before the loss. Do you really want that alternately grouchy slug with the pot belly plunked back in the easy chair, asking when dinner's going to be ready? I doubt it. Be happy that he's doing what he's doing—and that you played a major role in his transformation. You can't expect him to change his physical being and remain the same person—especially relative to exercise. And, as with the Romeo phase, I find that most men moderate their habits after a few months and cut back their running, weight lifting and other physical activities to a more reasonable level. Since you will probably take up some of his activities, you can meet somewhere in the middle.

YOUR POSITION IN YOUR "NEW" RELATIONSHIP

Remember that you are starting this new phase with your man in a very advantageous position. You are the heroine, having helped him through a difficult stage, and in my experience, even if your man does run off to the track with his buddies every evening, he will recognize (but don't expect him to admit it), that you are the most important person in his life.

On the other hand—and this relates to our discussion about his tendency to flirt and overindulge in sports—you'll have to be a little more careful about your attitude toward him. He'll no longer be the moody, overweight guy who comes home to the same chair and swings the refrigerator door open at the same time every night. You'll no longer be able to take him or his behavior for granted, and that element of surprise should be the first step in your constructing a new relationship together.

SARAH VERDON

It was difficult, at first, after my John lost the 60 pounds the doctor told him had to go. We were both surprised at how we'd begun to lead separate lives, because his weight was making *both* of us unhappy. So when it finally came off, we didn't know quite where to start.

We had a talk together about it, and we decided to seek out activities that we could do together. Not things that were really designed for one, with one of us tagging along after the other, but things designed for couples. And I made sure that as many as possible were active and involved other active people. Now, John's a CPA and I'm a bank branch manager, which are pretty stiff jobs, but you know what we went crazy over? Ballroom dancing. I know it sounds kind of corny, but it's romantic, it's great exercise, and it's *together*, which is my favorite part.

The couples who I've seen make it work best after a man's weight loss worked toward striking a balance between health and romance. Ballroom dancing, to me, is a terrific example of what I mean. But make your own choice.

TOGETHER IN HEALTH

What I've tried to do throughout this book is to help bring you and your man closer together on a variety of levels. Helping get him into shape accomplishes just that. Or, at the very least, it gets both of you out of the rut that poor health can land you in. Depression gives way to happiness, togetherness, and a renewal of the friendship and romance you remember from the beginning of your relationship. That should be a primary goal of your campaign to help him.

ANNA WILLIAMSON

We really went through a wonderful transformation after I helped Alex get into shape, and more than that, after he got *used* to being in shape and accepted himself as a thinner person. I have to confess that I actually had some problems adjusting to some of the personality changes he started experiencing and that seemed to arrive with his new body—there was a little bit of swaggering at first. But then I learned to appreciate it—in bed and out of it. We both rediscovered the fact that we liked to have good sex together and we liked to talk together, and even though he's gotten to be something of an exercise nut and overdoes it sometimes, I notice it less. Mostly because I've actually gotten into better shape by going along with him on 10K runs and hiking trips. We made a pact: one weekend we do what he wants, the next we do what I want.

In my mind—and remember I started him on the whole thing—the most important thing that's come out of this is the fact that Alex's health is much better and his self-esteem is improved—not to mention the savings in our weekly grocery bill. But it was our life as a couple that really changed. There's a *oneness* between us now that we hadn't had since we first started living together.

And that wonderful feeling, shared by two people who care about each other, is, in the end, what good health—and this book—are all about.

A FINAL WORD

When I made a choice to specialize in bariatric medicine over twenty years ago, I had decided that the American way of eating—and life—should change drastically, and at all levels and for all people: working class, middle class, upper class, black, white (Asians tend to eat more healthfully), gay, and straight—I was just interested in restoring people to health.

Two decades later, I'm no less of a health nut, but I am a little more of a realist about people (especially men) and their eating habits—what's possible and what's not—and I hope you are, too, now that you've read some of my stories.

What do I want you to take away from *How to Help Your Man Lose Weight*? First, the ability to help your man get down to a manageable size. Second, an awareness of how differently men and women are taught to view food in this country and how differently the sexes are treated when they're overweight. The concept of weight in America with its almost exclusive emphasis on women, reflects inequities between the sexes in politics and society as a whole. We have to understand that just as women are perfectly qualified to hold high office, men are perfectly capable of getting fat. Third, I'd like to believe that the knowledge that you've gained about your man's habits will help you in your own pursuit of health.

Lastly, and most of all, I'd like to think that you can spread the good-health gospel yourself, to as many of those among your family, friends, and loved ones (and maybe even a stranger or two) as you possibly can. In a society that suffers from as much overweight as does ours, when we reach the point where we can talk honestly about weight—and help one another do something about it—you'd be surprised at how many other problems will come into perspective as well.